WIND SPORTS

WIND SPORTS

By

ANABEL DEAN

THE WESTMINSTER PRESS

Philadelphia

BOOK DESIGN BY DOROTHY ALDEN SMITH

First edition

Published by The Westminster Press®
Philadelphia, Pennsylvania

PRINTED IN THE UNITED STATES OF AMERICA
9 8 7 6 5 4 3 2 1

CREDITS: *The Facts of Flight,* by Jerry Grey, pp. 24, 25, 26, 56; Manta Products, p. 55; Don Monroe, pp. 28, 29; NASA, pp. 33, 114, 115; Official U.S. Navy Photograph, pp. 120, 122, 123, 125, 126; The Science Museum, London, p. 36; Smithsonian Institution, pp. 15, 18, 22, 37, 38, 40, 43, 45, 67, 72, 75, 87, 90 (Ruth Law Oliver), 91; Greg Trott, p. 157; United Press International, pp. 58, 60, 144, 145; U.S. Forest Service, p. 117; George Uveges, pp. 30, 54; all others, Anabel Dean.

Library of Congress Cataloging in Publication Data

Dean, Anabel.
  Wind sports.

  Bibliography: p.
  Includes index.
  SUMMARY: Discusses the history, scientific principles, and practical and recreational uses of a variety of sports that utilize the wind in the air and on land, water, and ice.
  1. Gliding and soaring—Juvenile literature.
2. Parachuting—Juvenile literature. 3. Iceboating—Juvenile literature. 4. Windsurfing—Juvenile literature. 5. Sand yachts—Juvenile literature.
6. Sailing—Juvenile literature. [1. Gliding.
2. Parachuting. 3. Iceboating. 4. Windsurfing.
5. Sand yachts. 6. Sailing] I. Title.
GV764.D42 1982   797   82–13460
ISBN 0–664–32696–X

CONTENTS

Continued

An Invitation

The wind was the first force harnessed by humans to work for them. When people first went to sea, the wind pushed their boats along. When the first farmers tired of grinding corn and wheat, wind was harnessed to do this work.

Today we rarely use the unlimited energy of the wind to work for us. We depend on the ever-diminishing supplies of fossil fuels to provide the energy we need. Someday fossil fuels will all be gone. Then we may come back to our first source of energy, the wind.

In the meantime, though we aren't using the energy of the wind for work, let's use it for play. Winter, summer, spring, or fall, the wind can be your partner in one of the exciting wind sports. It will furnish the energy to move you along in the air, on the water, on ice, or on land. So have fun! Come, play with the wind!

PART ONE /*GLIDING*

---

1. EARLY PIONEERS

SIR GEORGE CAYLEY

"You mean, sir, you want me to lie down on that thing?" The coachman was puzzled. He knew that his employer, Sir George Cayley, was a little odd. As the old man was now eighty, the coachman put it down to old age.

"Yes, my good man. Just lie down on the fuselage, that is this part, and hold on here over the wing. You will go down in history as the first man to fly in a heavier-than-air craft."

The coachman knew there was no way that thing could fly. So, in order to humor the old man, he lay down on the glider as directed.

Sir George had positioned the glider on the brow of a hill. To it he had tied a long towrope. A little way down the hill another of his employees waited on horseback. Sir George carried the rope to him and had him wrap it firmly around the saddle horn.

When all was ready, Sir George yelled, "Go!"

The rider whipped up the horse. The glider gave a lurch. Then the startled coachman saw the grass receding below him. It took a few seconds for him to realize that he was actually flying. He was terrified as the glider flew several hundred feet through the air before it came safely back to rest again in the meadow.

The coachman quickly scrambled to his feet, afraid the glider would take him back up into the air. Sir George came puffing up. He was ecstatic.

"It flew, it flew!" he cried. "I knew it would. You will go down in history as the first man to fly in a heavier-than-air craft. Tomorrow I'll get two horses. I'm sure the glider can fly farther."

"Please, Sir George," said the coachman. "I wish to give notice. I was hired to drive your horses, not fly through the air."

The coachman was as good as his word. He never flew again. Evidently Sir George was unable to persuade any of his other employees to become a pilot in his place.

This first flight of a human in a heavier-than-air craft was made in 1853. It was made in the second full-size glider built by Sir George Cayley.

Sir George Cayley is considered the true father of aviation. Born in 1773, he was an Englishman and a Yorkshire baronet. From childhood he was fascinated by flight, and he devoted his life to trying to solve its riddle.

When George Cayley was a boy, Europe was seized with balloon fever. Everyone was fascinated with traveling through the air in lighter-than-air craft. But a few people believed that the future of flight would be in heavier-than-air craft. Most of these would-be flyers pinned their hopes on machines with flapping wings modeled after birds. Sir George Cayley felt that the shape of the wings would provide lift. Power would come from a lightweight engine.

By 1799, George Cayley had laid out the basic shape of today's airplane. His plans included fixed wings, which could be stacked up to make biplanes and triplanes. A flying machine, he decided, should have a long fuselage. Steering could be accomplished by elevators in the tail section to control the up and down movements and a rudder to turn right or left. The cycle wheel, invented by Sir

10

George, could be used to permit a glider to roll on the ground before and after flights. This wheel was the one adopted for use on airplanes.

By 1804, Cayley was making and flying model gliders. His experiments with these led him to publish his research on aerodynamics—the science of the way air affects a body in motion. Two of Sir George's findings laid the foundation for future experiments in flying. These were—

1. When a body moves through the air, a region of low pressure is generated that results in lift on the upper surface of the wing.
2. Streamlining permits a body to move through the air with less drag or resistance.

Sir George built two full-size gliders. The second one was as large as a World War II fighter. This glider, which made several short hops with a man on board, was the first one to fly. The inventor's advanced age, at this time, kept him from flying himself. Sir George invented everything needed for manned flight. But he also realized that no engine then in use was light enough to power an airplane. Powered flight would have to wait for the development of the internal-combustion engine.

JEAN-MARIE LE BRIS

The next person to get a glider into the air was Jean-Marie Le Bris. He was a Breton sea captain with a passion for flying. In 1856 he built a glider shaped like an albatross, with 23-foot wings. The body was boat-shaped.

Glider pilots in 1856 had one serious problem. Before a glider will fly, it must be moving at flying speed. This is the speed at which lift overcomes the force of gravity. Today gliders are usually towed behind an airplane to achieve that speed. In 1856 they were usually launched into the wind. Wind speed was substituted for flying speed. More of the gliders built at that time would probably have flown if there had been a better way to generate enough speed.

Captain Le Bris put his glider on a horse-drawn cart at the top of a rise on the coast of France. His invention must have been based on good aerodynamic principles. When the horse trotted downhill, the glider took off and flew 300 feet before landing. In 1868, Le Bris launched his glider again. This time he crashed and broke his leg.

In the nineteenth century there were two paths leading toward heavier-than-air manned flight. Those inventors who went with powered flight—in those days heavy steam engines—took one path. Those who concentrated on gliding flight took the path that eventually led to understanding aerodynamics. For years the huffers and puffers held the center stage without any real results. The gliders, on the other hand, were gathering flight experience and pioneering the science of aerodynamics. When the internal-combustion engine was perfected, they were ready to take advantage of it.

OTTO LILIENTHAL

Gliders and hang gliders have many of the same pioneers and heroes. Since Otto Lilienthal is considered the father of hang gliding, he is included in that section. But the contributions he made to gliding are so important that he will be referred to from time to time in this section.

OCTAVE CHANUTE

Octave Chanute was born in France in 1832. Since his parents moved to the United States when he was six, he was educated here. In time he became a well-known bridge engineer. At that time, most people regarded anyone interested in flying as a visionary and a dreamer—certainly lacking in common sense. For that reason, although Chanute had a lifelong interest in flying, he kept it a secret. But he kept records and investigated every flying experiment he heard about. Soon Octave Chanute was the leading authority on flying machines. In 1891 a friend persuaded him to write a history of these experiments as a curiosity. Seizing upon this excuse, Chanute wrote *Progress in Flying Machines,* which detailed all experiments made to that date.

In 1896, although well over sixty, Octave Chanute decided that the time had come to devote all his energies to the problem of the flying machine. Chanute and a group of assistants began to make experiments with gliders on the sand dunes of Lake Michigan. Chanute was searching for

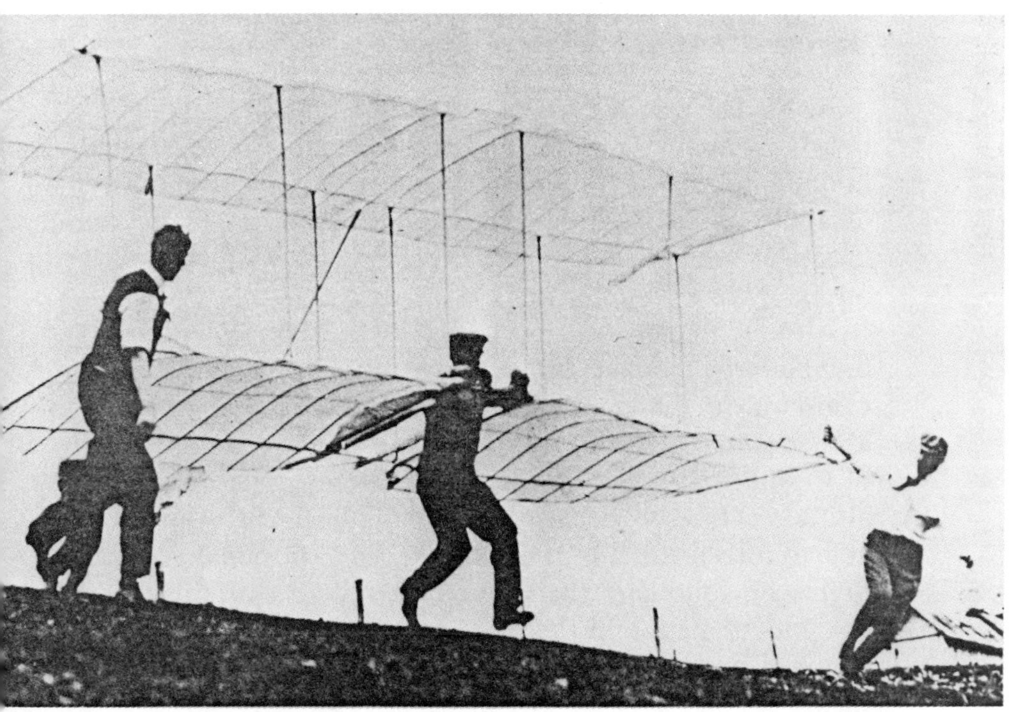

The AEA Chanute type of hang glider being launched at Hammondsport, New York, winter 1907–08

a better way to control a glider in flight. In Europe, Otto Lilienthal had been guiding a hang glider by swinging his body. Chanute felt there must be a better way to steer a glider.

Chanute and his group made over two hundred flights with five different types of gliders. Careful records were kept and photographs made of all experiments. Their most successful flights were made using a biplane with a rudder and wings segmented—divided into parts. Chanute became a close friend and correspondent of Wilbur and Orville Wright, who were to make the first successful powered flight. He was their adviser and visited them at least once at Kitty Hawk.

AUGUSTUS MOORE HERRING

A. M. Herring was one of the men associated with Octave Chanute in designing and building gliders. He assisted in designing some of their most successful craft. For a time Chanute became discouraged and withdrew from the group. When this happened, Herring decided to strike out on his own.

Although hampered by a lack of money, Herring did build a large triplane glider. Flight-tested at Chanute's old camp on the dunes, the glider was a success. Herring was able to make glides of up to 927 feet—twice as far as any of Chanute's gliders had traveled. At times he flew at an altitude of from 40 to 50 feet. Herring, for the first time, was able to turn the glider in the air. He learned to make longer flights by following the curve of a hill to ride the rising currents of air found there. About this time, though, Herring ran out of money and had to discontinue his experiments.

After searching for backing for some time, Herring got Matthias Arnot to finance some of his experiments. Herring

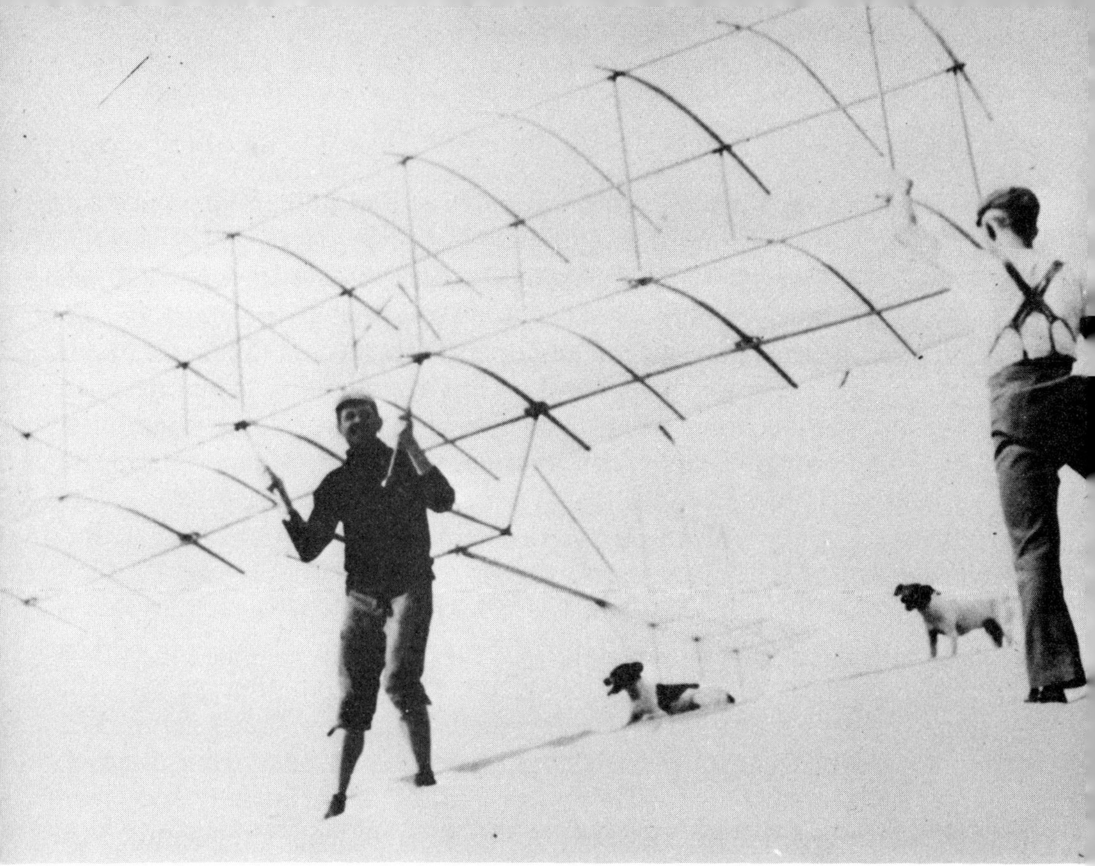

A. M. Herring's biplane glider barely hopped above the ground

now built a biplane glider. Later, he mounted an engine in this glider. In it he was able to make two short hops about a yard above the ground. But he was never able to make a sustained flight.

THE WRIGHT BROTHERS

Wilbur Wright was born in 1867, his brother, Orville, in 1871. The boys were lifelong companions. They lived, thought, and worked together and are always mentioned together. Neither one of them ever claimed credit for any invention without including the other. At an early age both boys showed excellent mechanical ability. They were born tinkers and inventors. While still in their teens, they designed a paper-folding machine and built a large printing press.

In 1892, Wilbur and Orville became interested in the safety-bicycle craze that was sweeping the country. Together they opened and operated a successful bicycle manufacturing and repair shop in Dayton, Ohio. The boys were industrious, frugal, and friendly. Their shop prospered. It provided them with an income, tools, equipment, and mechanical knowledge. It gave them background and income so they could pursue other mechanical interests that were more challenging to them.

In 1896, the subject of manned flight was of interest to everyone in the United States. Every newspaper carried accounts and pictures of the experiments then going on. It was natural that the problems of flight should capture Wilbur's and Orville's imagination. Both boys were intensely interested in Otto Lilienthal's experiments and were touched by his death in a glider accident. They combed the local libraries and bookstores for material on flight, with little success. In 1899, Wilbur wrote to the Smithsonian Institution asking for a list of books and articles on flying. The Smithsonian sent reprints of articles and a list of books. Soon, one of these books, Chanute's *Progress in Flying Machines,* became their basic text. The young men were now able to study the work of others interested in flying. But they soon found that aeronautical theory of that time was a mass of conflicting ideas and guesswork. It offered little for a newcomer to build upon. But they were able to dig some useful information out of the material. Lilienthal had published the air-pressure tables he had used in planning the wing surfaces of his gliders. The brothers felt that Lilienthal's success in flying hang gliders proved the accuracy of these tables. Wilbur and Orville also felt that the biplane models, or two-surface machines, of Chanute and Herring were the most promising. Both felt that the biggest problem of aviation was the control of the machine. Although the

16

two brothers had little formal education, their intensive studies soon transformed them into scientists dedicated to solving the problems of flight.

From his observation of birds, Wilbur concluded that birds controlled their flight by twisting, or warping, their wings. He decided that warping could be used to control a glider. In August 1899, the two men built a biplane kite with a 5-foot wingspan. They used it to experiment with the control of lifting surfaces. This kite was fitted with wires by which the wings could be warped during flight.

By now Wilbur and Orville had decided that control and stability in the air could best be accomplished by fastening the two wings of a biplane glider together with wires. This would, they hoped, enable them to twist the wings to bank and turn. Their first glider, with a 17-foot wingspan, was built on this plan.

The men did some research to find the best place from which to launch a glider. They chose Kitty Hawk, North Carolina, because of the strong prevailing winds there. The sand dunes, which would be soft for landing, and the isolation all added up to make this an ideal site. In September 1900, they took their glider there. First it was tested as an unmanned kite. Then Wilbur lay on the bottom wing and held on. Orville took the strong line and ran down the sand dune. The kite rose into the air and glided for a few feet. But attempts to fly this glider in free flight were disappointing. The men went back to Dayton on October 22, confused and dissatisfied.

Back in Dayton, Wilbur and Orville set to work building a large glider with a 22-foot wingspan. They felt that their first model had not had a large enough wing surface. In July 1901, they took this model to Kitty Hawk to be tested. The men made many flights with this glider that summer. But although number 2, as this glider was called, flew as far as three hundred feet, it was erratic in the air. Control was a problem. It was at this time that Octave Chanute came to

17

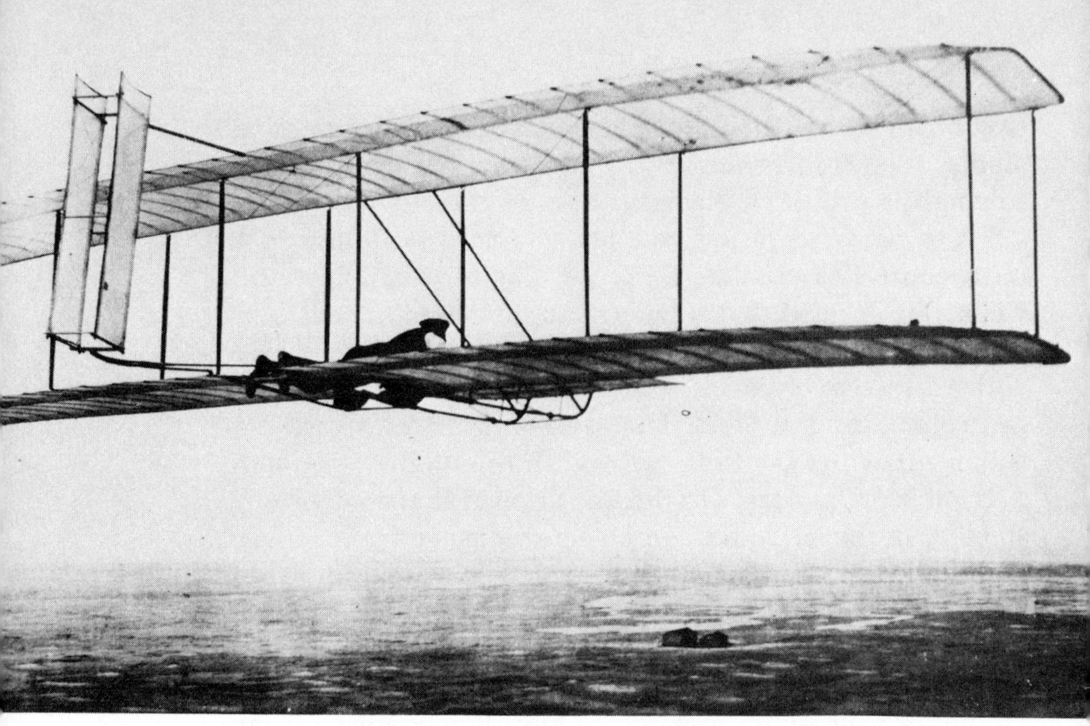

Orville Wright flying the brothers' 1902 glider

visit them at Kitty Hawk and photographed number 2 in flight.

When Wilbur and Orville went back to Dayton for the winter, they were both discouraged. Their machine, besides being erratic, couldn't fly unless there was a brisk wind. Both men felt that the published data on air lift and drag, which they had been using, were inaccurate. The lift on their glider was only one third of that predicted by the tables. At this point the brothers became true scientists. They built two wind tunnels and tested over two hundred designs for wings and propellers. Then they became engineers and used the information they had gathered to design a new glider. In August and September 1902, they built glider number 3. It had a 32-foot wingspan and incorporated all the findings from their experiments. This glider had one control, which operated the movable tail and the warping of the wings.

18

In September 1903, Wilbur and Orville were back at Kitty Hawk to test number 3. Things at last seemed to be going their way. Some adjustments and changes were found to be necessary on their new glider. But that summer the two men made over one thousand glides in this machine. Some of these flights were as long as six hundred feet. The stability and control problems had all been solved. It was the first effectively controlled glider in history.

In the meantime, technology was catching up with the flying machine. The development of a small internal-combustion gasoline engine for use in automobiles had provided lightweight power. The Wright brothers, however, could not find the engine they needed. Their next step was to build an engine of the right size, weight, and power. It was a 4-cylinder gasoline engine. When they put that engine in a biplane of their own design and added a propeller, the rest was history.

The Wright brothers did not give up gliders after their first powered flight. Wilbur continued to study gliding and soaring. In 1911, to test his theories, the brothers again built a glider. This new one was equipped with more powerful controls. With the new controls and a horizontal rudder on the tail, the brothers made some long glides. The longest, 9 minutes and 45 seconds, was made in 1911. This remained a world record for ten years.

But, except for the Wright brothers, interest in gliding almost ceased from 1910 to 1920. Powered flight captured the imagination of the world, until after World War I, when clauses in the Treaty of Versailles caused the Germans to take a new look at gliders.

GLIDERS IN GERMANY AFTER WORLD WAR I

World War I caused the Allies to distrust Germany's interest in airplanes. The Treaty of Versailles denied them the use of powered aircraft. The result was a renewed interest in gliding. That, and the fact that the air currents in the Rhine valley are ideal for soaring, soon made Germany a leader in gliding.

The first glider competition was held in the Rhön Mountains in 1920. The best performance then was a flight of 6,000 feet in 2½ minutes. But on August 30, 1921, a German, Wolfgang Klemperer, soared over the Rhine valley for 13 minutes and broke the record held by the Wright brothers.

By 1922, Germany was building and flying true sailplanes. These were not like the heavier, cruder machines previously used for gliding. They were almost like the ones in use today. With their long slender wings and enclosed cockpits, they were almost perfect aerodynamically.

The Germans, by 1928, were doing what they called cloud soaring. They were using upcurrents of air under cumulus clouds to achieve altitude and to lengthen flying time. In 1929, two German glider pilots invented the variometer, an instrument now used in all gliders to indicate whether an aircraft is rising or sinking.

Gliding in Germany, at this period, was at first done as a sport. But it soon became a means of training pilots for future *Luftwaffe* squadrons. German scientists used gliders to study aerodynamics and the efficient use of lightweight materials. The knowledge gained proved extremely useful when Hitler chose to disregard the Treaty of Versailles in 1935. By 1939, Germany had 186,000 glider pilots. These became the backbone of Germany's air force in World War II.

2. SOARING TODAY

WHAT KEEPS A SOARER UP?

Leonardo da Vinci bent forward to darken the shadows under the trees in his painting. A shadow passed over the canvas. Leonardo looked up to see a hawk circling overhead.

The painting was forgotten. The paint dried on the palette as the man stared, fascinated. How smoothly and gracefully the bird soared! Its wings were motionless. Leonardo da Vinci wondered, as he had many times before, why humans couldn't fly like birds.

Leonardo laid down his brush. Of course, people could fly. All they had to do was build wings. Then they too could soar.

Leonardo picked up paper and pencil and began drawing. From time to time, he glanced up at the birds still circling overhead. When he had finished, hours later, Leonardo had drawn plans for a flying machine. His sketch was of a machine with flapping wings modeled after those of a bird. It should be built of lightweight materials. Ropes and pulleys would be used so the flyer could flap the wings. Perhaps, he thought, I will be the first man to defy earth's gravity and fly.

This was around 1505. As far as is known, no one ever

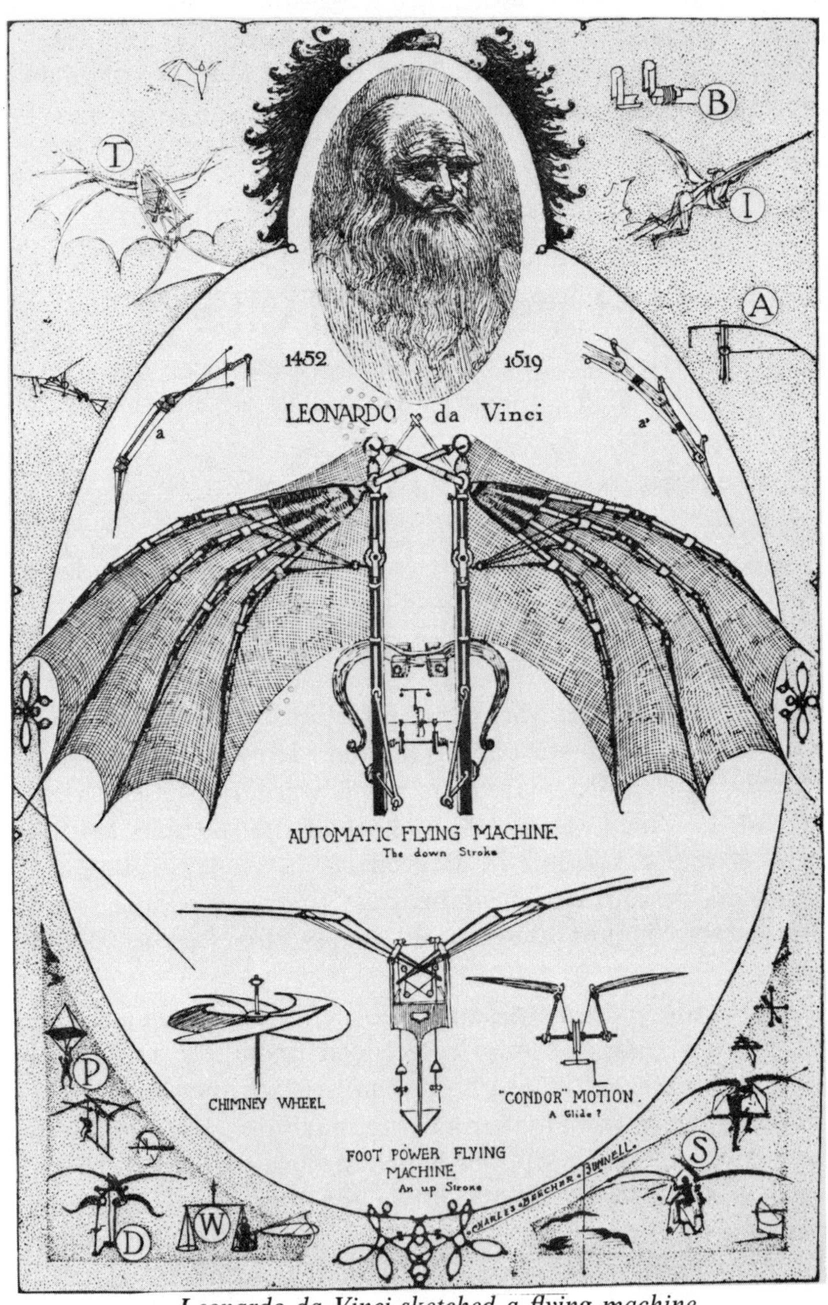

*Leonardo da Vinci sketched a flying machine
almost five centuries ago*

built or tried to fly Leonardo's model. But many people since have tried to build flying machines with flapping wings. Leonardo, and many others after him, overestimated the strength and endurance of human muscles. No one has ever been able to flap a pair of wings fast enough to get off the ground.

Have you ever watched a hawk circling high overhead, the way Leonardo da Vinci did five hundred years ago? The hawk is soaring. It does not need to flap its wings, because it has found a source of lift—a column of rising air. Have you ever wished that you could soar like a hawk? For centuries people have wished to do this, without knowing how it could be done. But today we know how. You too can soar!

Did you notice we said soar? There is a difference between soaring and gliding. A soarer is riding an updraft of air. A glider is always descending.

Gliders were the forerunners of the true soarers—the sailplanes. The early pioneers of powerless flight all built and operated gliders. Their machines, after takeoff, were at all times gliding downward to an eventual landing. Any heavier-than-air craft must move forward to stay aloft. If it stops, it goes into a stall and falls. Powered aircraft use an engine to keep them moving forward; gliders use the force of gravity. Gravity causes gliders to coast downhill through an invisible sea of air.

All gliders, or sailplanes, as they are now usually called, have a glide ratio, or sinking speed. This is the maximum distance the craft can travel forward for every foot of altitude it loses in still air. Design and weight have a lot to do with flying efficiency. Early gliders traveled only a couple of feet forward for every foot they descended. Today the ultralight, streamlined sailplanes with extra-long wings have very low sinking speeds. The best competition sailplanes can travel almost fifty feet forward for every foot they lose in altitude. Most of the modern sailplanes have a

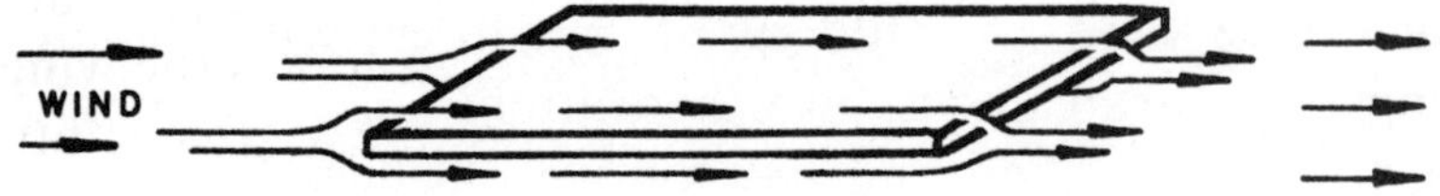

*Point a board directly windward and no forces
act except a slight drag*

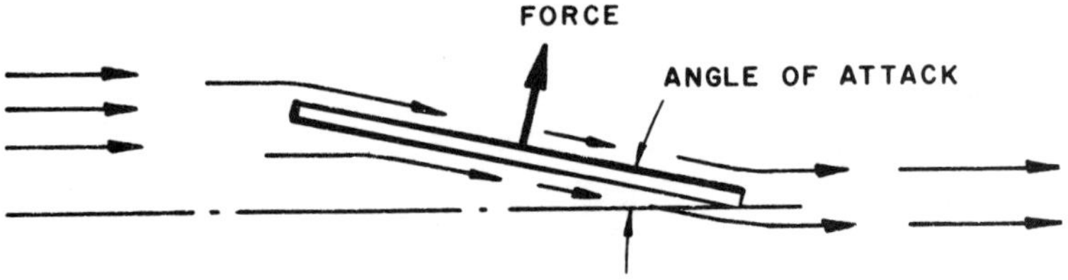

Tilt the board at an angle and a lift force results

glide ratio of about 26 to 1.

This is all very well. But what keeps a sailplane up in the first place? Why doesn't it just fall down? To understand this you must know a little about aerodynamics, or how air affects a body in motion. One principle is basic to all aviation. That is Bernoulli's principle, which states that the pressure of a fluid or gas decreases when the speed of either one increases. To find out how this principle works, let's look at the wings of an aircraft. The first thing to notice is that they are not of uniform thickness. The front edge is always thicker than the rear edge. The top side of the wing is always curved—the underside always flat. This design forms what is known as an airfoil. When the plane is in motion, air is split by the leading edge of the wing. Part of the air goes up and over the curved upper surface of the wing. The rest goes past the flat underside of the wing. The air passing over the curved upper section must travel a greater distance than that going over the flat underside. The air on top travels faster to catch up with the air traveling over the lower surface. Following Bernoulli's principle, this

24

reduces the pressure on the top of the wing. As the pressure on the bottom of the wing is then greater, it forces the wing up and produces lift. A faster speed produces greater lift. This lift keeps an airplane or sailplane in the air.

LIFT

Now we have seen that a sailplane can glide steadily downward without falling to earth. But what provides the lift to enable it to climb and soar? The sailplane pilot depends on currents of air to carry the plane higher.

Ridge Lift

The ridge lift was the first lift discovered by glider pilots. When the prevailing wind strikes a hill, cliff, or ridge, it is deflected upward. If the wind is strong, the air current will rise several hundred feet above the ridge. A steady wind provides ideal soaring conditions. A pilot can fly back and forth in a ridge lift for hours. Flights of over a thousand miles have been made by following a ridge lift along a chain

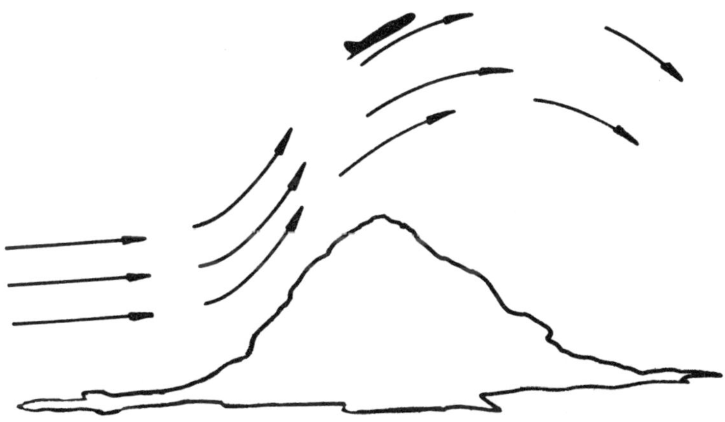

Wind striking the side of a hill produces an upward current

of mountains. Spectacular soaring conditions are produced when the prevailing wind off the ocean strikes a high cliff. The sea cliffs at Torrey Pines near San Diego are a famous soaring spot.

Thermal

A column of rising warm air, called a thermal, offers a different type of soaring. Although not as long-lived as ridge lifts, thermals often lift a sailplane higher. Thermals are caused by the sun heating the earth to different temperatures. For that reason, thermals are found only when there is some sunshine. Rocks, plowed fields, large stretches of asphalt, and bare land absorb heat and reflect it upward.

The sailplane pilot has one problem when seeking a thermal. The rising air can't be seen. A person learns from experience where thermals are located. Sometimes circling birds indicate one. When riding thermals, the pilot circles until that thermal has carried the plane as high as possible. Then the pilot glides to the next likely-looking spot. If the pilot is both lucky and skillful, he or she can put together a chain of updrafts. The variometer is necessary when riding thermals. It tells the pilot when he or she has found a thermal and helps locate the spot where lift is greatest.

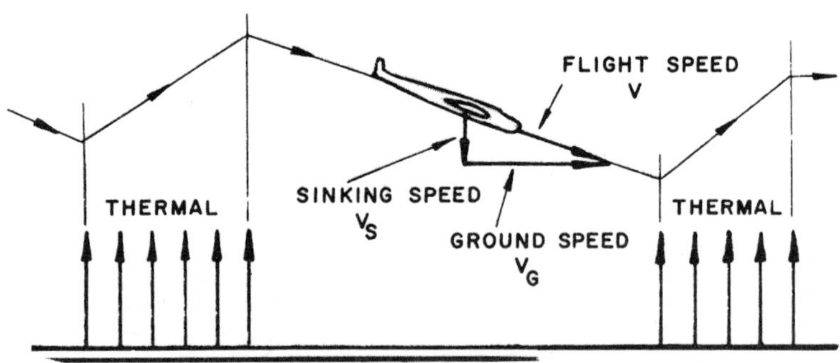

*A plane sinks between thermals and the pilot
must catch the next thermal to stay aloft*

Lee Wave or Mountain Wave

Lee waves or mountain waves provide the most exciting soaring conditions. A mountain wave occurs when a stream of fast-moving air strikes a mountain, blows over it and down the other side. The air then strikes the stable air near the ground and bounces back up into another wave. Usually there are several waves in succession. This same effect can be seen in a stream when the water flows over a submerged boulder. Several smaller waves will lie downstream from the boulder. Mountain waves provide greater lift than other updrafts of air. One pilot, Paul F. Bikle, flew to an altitude of almost 9 miles in one of these waves. Of course, protective clothing and oxygen are necessary for flights to high altitudes.

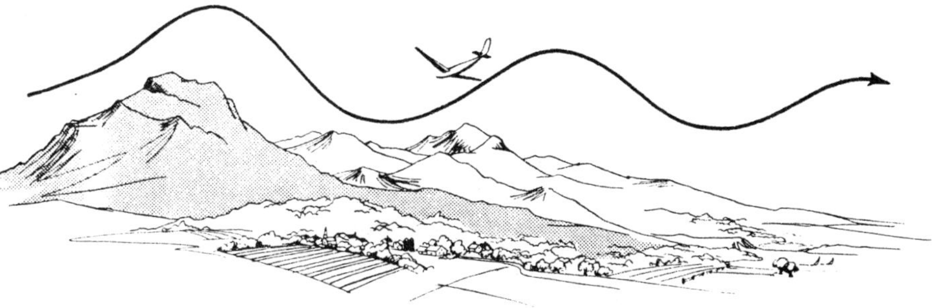

Riding the lee wave

WHO CAN FLY A SAILPLANE?

The answer to that question is, almost anyone. A physical examination isn't even necessary. Fourteen is the minimum age for flight instruction. But ground instruction is available for younger students. There is no upper age limit. Recently a retired teacher made his first solo glider flight at the age of eighty-two.

If you are reading this book, you probably are interested in soaring. But think twice about it. It isn't as inexpensive

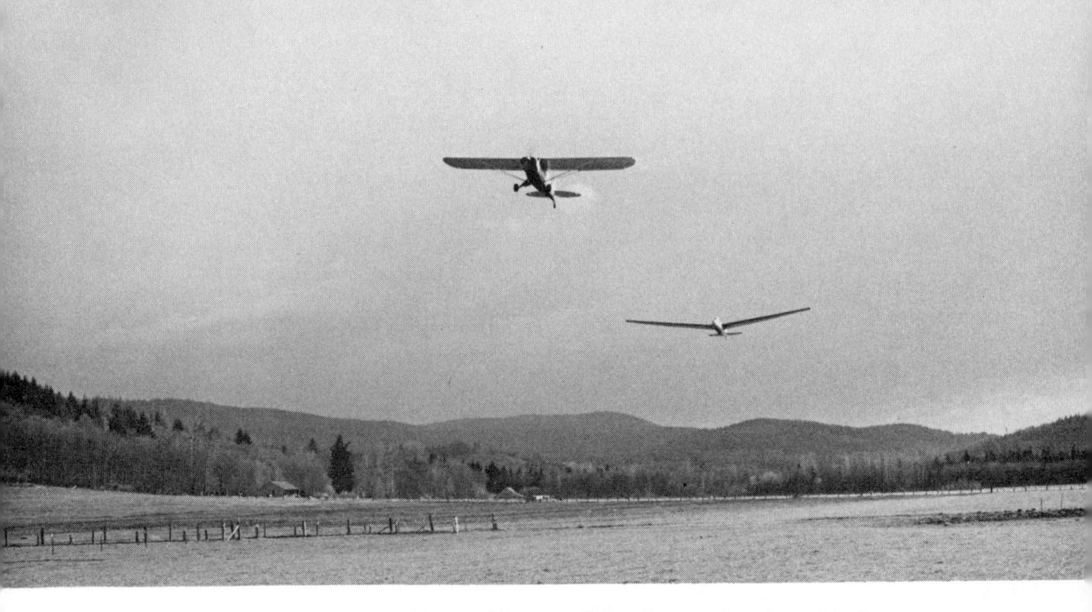

Launching a glider by towing it behind an airplane

as are many sports. Before you put out any money for lessons, go out to a glider port and observe the action. Watch the gliders take off and land. Talk to the people. You will find them friendly and enthusiastic. If you like what you see and hear, you are ready to take a ride in a sailplane. Most glider ports, especially those offering lessons, give introductory rides in a two-seated training plane. If, after a ride, you are still interested in gliding, sign up for lessons with a reputable sailplane school. No book can teach you how to pilot a glider safely.

LAUNCHING THE GLIDER

Before it can fly, a glider must be accelerated to flying speed. At one time, gliders had such low flying speeds they could be launched into a brisk wind. Sailplanes today have a much higher flying speed. More speed is necessary. Most gliders in the United States are launched by being towed behind a small airplane. The speed and altitude provided by the airplane ensure a glide of at least twenty minutes, even if no updraft is found for additional lift.

Gliders are also launched by being towed behind an automobile. As the glider only attains an altitude of from 400 to 900 feet, the glide is much shorter. The greatest success with automobile towing occurs near ridges, or in the desert, where there is a strong lift near ground level.

Gliders are sometimes launched by a shock-cord launcher. This works something like a giant slingshot. The glider is "snapped off" a ridge or cliff. More common today is the motor-driven winch tow launcher. This works something like a giant fishing reel. The glider is reeled to the edge of the cliff like a fish on the end of a line. A glider can attain a speed of about 50 miles per hour and an altitude of from 500 to 1,500 feet with a winch tow. A small parachute is attached to the cable to keep it from snarling as it drops back to earth. Winch tow launching is less expensive than

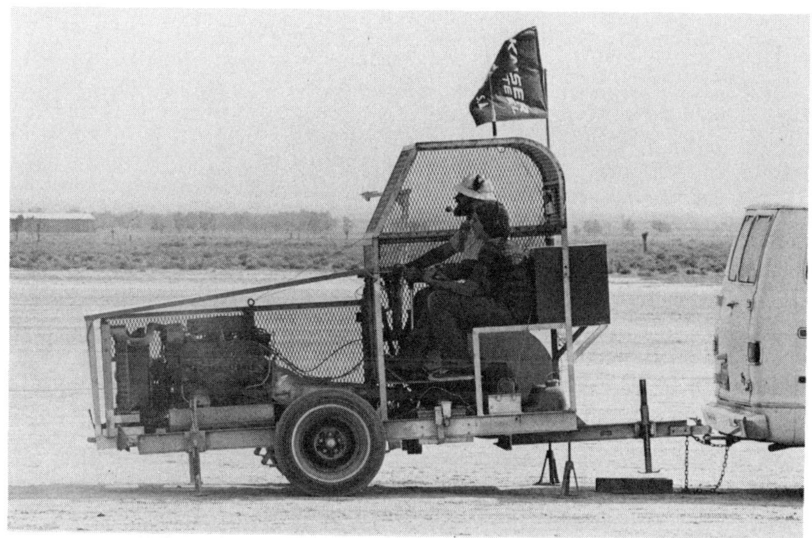

Controlling the shock-cord launcher

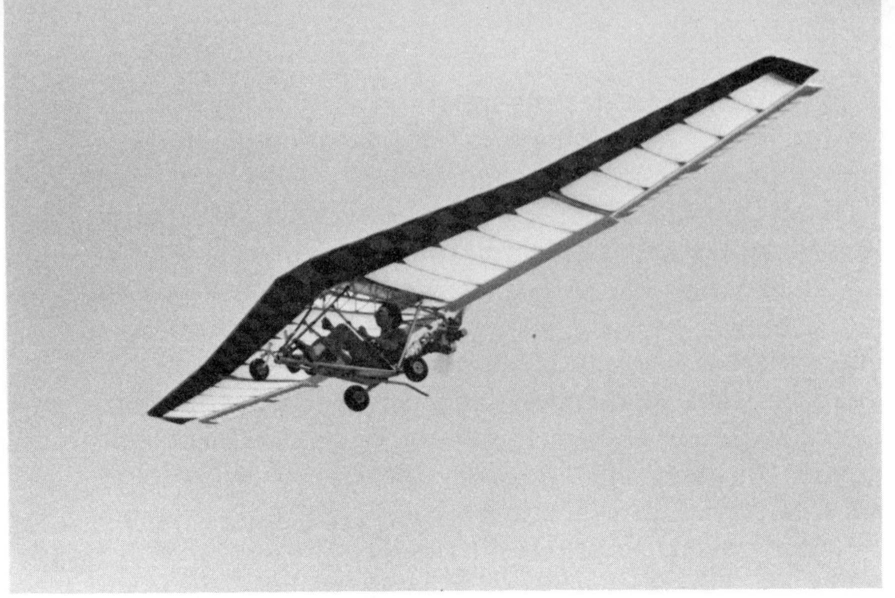

An ultralight glider

using a tow plane. But several people are still required to operate the winch.

Some gliders, known as ultralights, are now equipped with a small engine. The ultralight can take off on its own and fly to a thermal. There the engine is shut off and the ultralight becomes a glider. After a day of soaring, the pilot starts the engine and flies back to the port.

CROSS-COUNTRY SOARING

Most pilots only soar around home port. They get to know where the thermals in that area are located. The home glider port offers security when they run out of lift.

The more adventurous like to try cross-country soaring. Here the pilot of the sailplane goes wherever a thermal can be found. He or she has to plan where to go to look for a new thermal before leaving one. The object is to string together as many thermals as possible in order to travel as

30

far as possible. Cross-country hops of up to 700 miles have been made.

The cross-country soarer needs a ground crew. This usually consists of friends or members of the family. They follow along below, towing a trailer for the sailplane. Sometimes a two-way radio is used for communication. When the pilot can't find another thermal and has to land, the glider is disassembled. The wings can be quickly unbolted and taken off for trailering. Then the pilot and the glider ride back to the home port.

COMPETITION

Most soarers aren't interested in competition. They prefer to try to better their own records. Badges are given by the Soaring Society of America for staying aloft different lengths of time. The better pilots are always trying to break the records set by other pilots. But there are races and derbies. In these, sailplanes are divided into classes according to their glide ratio.

The Smirnoff Sailplane Derby is perhaps the most famous. The gliders race from Los Angeles to Dulles Airport in Washington, D.C.—a distance of 2,900 miles. This is a stage race. The object is not to fly the distance at one time. Contestants fly in legs of from two hundred to three hundred miles each day. The pilots received points for speed and distance covered on each leg. The pilot who accumulates the most points is the winner.

PRACTICAL USES FOR GLIDERS

From the earliest days of aviation, gliders have been an important tool in airplane development. A machine that flies without an engine must be carefully designed. After World War I, Germany began to train airplane pilots in gliders. Even today in Europe, gliders are used in many pilot-training programs. Because there is no engine, pilots start out with fewer things to worry about. They learn how an aircraft flies without an engine to depend on.

In World War II gliders went to war. Germany began building large gliders for use as troop transports. These gliders did no soaring. They were made into trains and pulled along by transport planes. In May 1940, the Germans used trains of gliders in their attacks on Belgium, the Netherlands, and Luxembourg. Each glider carried 6 fully armed soldiers. Belgian forts were conquered by attacks of glider-carried troops.

In May 1941, Germany attacked the island of Crete, then held by Great Britain. The Germans landed nearly twenty-three thousand men with parachutes and in gliders to defeat the British.

Military men in the United States learned a lesson from Germany's use of gliders. They too began to build and use large gliders. Some of these plywood gliders were large enough to carry thirty infantrymen, a jeep, and a light field gun. Thousands of Allied troops were landed by gliders behind the beachheads in Normandy on D-day.

The glider became a valuable meteorological tool from 1935 on. Because of the slower speed and lack of vibration, delicate instruments operated better on a glider than on an airplane. Sailplanes were found to be the ideal vehicle from which to study thunderstorms. Slow-flying gliders, equipped with radio and recording instruments, could ride a thermal right up into a thunderhead.

In 1950 and 1951, the U.S. Air Force used gliders to

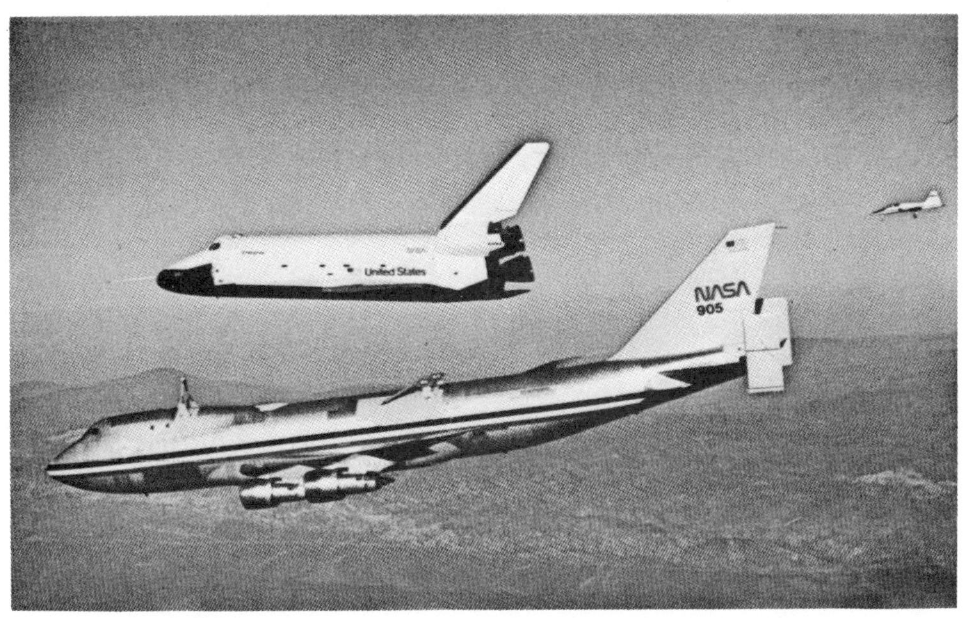

The spacecraft Enterprise, *like the* Columbia,
is a glider

study the flow of air over the Sierra Nevada. During these studies, Lawrence Edgar and Harold Klieforth established a high-altitude record. A mountain wave carried them to an altitude of 44,255 feet. This record was later broken by Paul F. Bikle.

Gliders also have a role in the space age. The spacecraft *Columbia* is a glider. Rockets are used to boost it into space. It uses maneuvering engines for positioning. But when it comes to landing, *Columbia* glides back down to earth the way any glider does.

---

3. EARLY HANG GLIDERS

DAEDALUS AND ICARUS

Long ago, on the island of Crete, there lived a sculptor and architect of extraordinary talent. Daedalus built a labyrinth, or maze, under the palace of the ruler, Minos. This labyrinth, the home of the monster, Minotaur, was so ingenious no one could escape from it without help. Daedalus also built a wooden cow that gave milk for Pasiphaë, Minos' wife. But his greatest creation was a bronze robot that fought and defeated the Argonauts, enemies of Minos.

Later, Minos became angry with Daedalus. He imprisoned the sculptor and his son, Icarus, in a tower on a rocky headland. The king kept a close watch on all departing ships so that the two men could not leave Crete.

"Minos may control the land and sea, but he doesn't control the regions of the air," Daedalus said. He set to work to build two pairs of wings. The sculptor made a mold to fit Icarus' arms and another to fit his own. Then he sewed feathers to the molds. The smaller feathers were stuck on with wax. The two men tried flapping these wings and found they could rise from the ground.

Before leaving to fly to Sicily, Daedalus cautioned Icarus. "Don't fly too low or the damp air of the sea will clog your feathers. Don't fly too high or the sun will melt the wax."

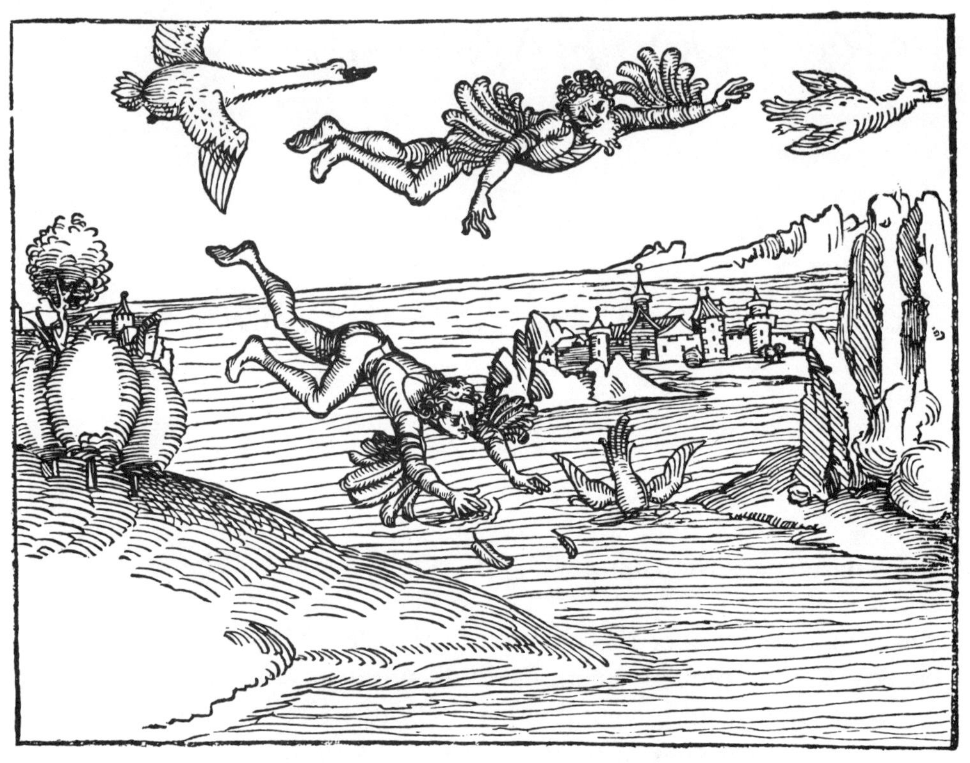

"The Flight of Daedalus and Fall of Icarus"

Daedalus and Icarus took off for Sicily. Icarus was intoxicated with the thrill of flying. Ignoring his father's cries and warnings, he flew higher and higher. Too late Icarus realized his mistake. The heat of the sun melted the wax and the feathers fell out. Icarus plunged into the sea and was never seen again.

Did Daedalus and Icarus really make this flight? Probably not—this is an old Greek myth. But, because humans have always yearned to fly like birds, there are many myths about flying. It wasn't until three thousand years later that people finally mastered the art of flying like birds. There have been as many downs as ups on this long road to flight. Icarus was the first man to fall from the skies; he was not the last.

36

Hang gliding and gliding have many of the same pioneers. In the early days an experimenter often built and flew both types of glider to test his theories. The only difference between a glider and a hang glider is the position of the pilot's body. In a hang glider, the pilot's body hangs down. Today's glider or sailplane has an enclosed cockpit. But on the early ones the pilot just lay or sat on the lower wing.

LOUIS MOUILLARD

Were all those early experimenters with hang gliders brave and daring? Well, it took a lot of courage for them to go up in the air. Some frankly admitted to being scared stiff. Louis Mouillard later wrote to Octave Chanute, "Goodness, how frightened I had been."

Louis Mouillard was born in Lyons, France, in 1835. As a young man he emigrated to Algeria. Like many of the other early flying enthusiasts, he was interested in the way birds flew. He wrote several articles on the subject. In the

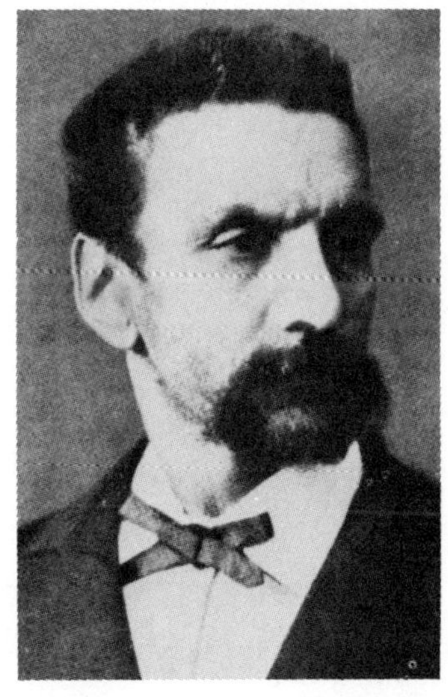

Louis Mouillard (1835–1897), glider inventor

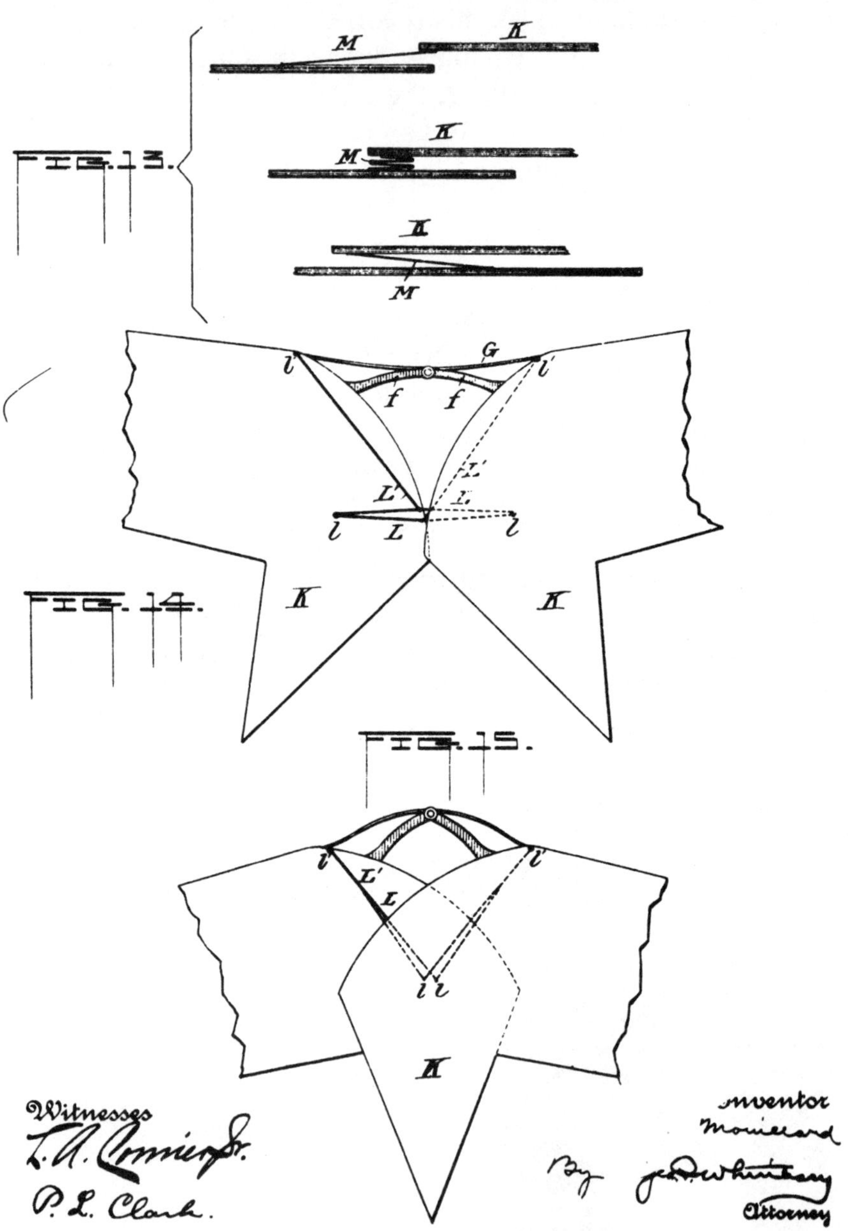

Sketch of Mouillard's hang glider

38

late 1850s Mouillard built three gliders. All the designs, as would be expected, were based on his study of birds. The third glider was just a pair of hinged wings fastened together in the center. These wings, constructed of curved agave sticks screwed to muslin-covered boards, were fastened to the shoulders of the pilot.

Very early one morning Louis Mouillard took his 33-pound hang glider out into the desert. He didn't want anyone to see him trying to fly. In those days anyone interested in flying was considered to be a little strange.

Mouillard strapped on his wings and looked around for a likely spot to try them. He was standing on a wagon road which had been raised five feet above the surrounding desert. There was a deep ditch on each side where dirt had been dug out to raise the road. Louis wanted to get across this ditch to the desert. As it wasn't very wide, he took a run and jumped.

He sailed easily over the ditch. "But, oh horrors," he said in his letter to Chanute, "once across the ditch my feet did not come down to earth!" Mouillard flew 138 feet. "But," as he said, "I was too terrified to enjoy the experience."

Later, Mouillard built other gliders that were not so successful. He also wrote a book, *L'Empire de l'Air,* about his experiments.

OTTO LILIENTHAL

It was still dark when Otto reached over and shook Gustav's shoulder. "We'd better get up now, Gus. It's almost daylight."

Gus, who was a year younger than Otto, shook off his brother's hand. He pulled the covers over his head and mumbled, "It's still dark. Let me sleep, Otto."

"All right," said Otto, who was already out of bed and groping for his clothes. "I'll go fly it myself."

"You wouldn't," said Gus doubtfully. He was peering out from under the covers now.

"I would," said Otto. He was already pulling on his boots.

"Wait for me, Otto." Gus jumped out of bed and, with chattering teeth, felt around for his clothes. "I'm coming."

Quietly the boys stole down the stairs from their attic bedroom. The farmhouse courtyard was lit by a faint gray light. Instinctively the two boys stopped and looked up at the chimney. A ragged pile was all that could be seen of the stork's nest that capped their chimney. All the chimneys in Pomerania were similarly capped. Now, silhouetted against the pearly-gray sky, the stork stood up. It looked ungainly as it stretched. Then it launched itself into the air.

The boys watched, fascinated, as the bird, clumsy on its feet, became a beautiful flying machine. This bird was the cause of the intense activity of Otto and Gus. They were

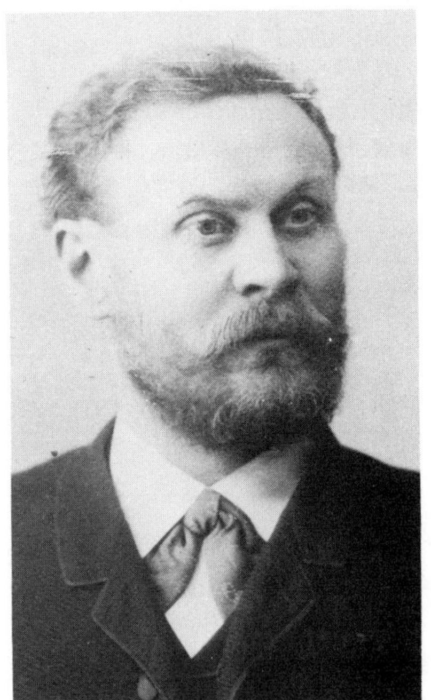

Otto Lilienthal (1848–1896), daring pioneer

determined to build a machine that could fly as did the stork. Already they had tried building small machines with flapping wings. Now they had finished a more ambitious one. It had fixed wings and would, they hoped, take one of them into the air. When the sun came up, there was always a strong breeze on a small hill near their home. This morning they intended to launch their glider from that hill.

The boys first visited a haystack some distance from the house. Here they had hidden their glider built with a framework of sticks and covered with brown paper. Together the boys carried it to the top of the hill.

When the sun peeked through a gap in the distant mountains, Otto was ready for takeoff. With Gus's help, he had tied on two birdlike wings. Now, when Otto felt the morning breeze on his face, he ran downhill, holding on to the wings. But he did not rise into the air as the stork had done. Instead, one wing caught against a bush. Otto went headfirst down the hill. A tangle of papers and sticks was all that was left of their glider.

This wasn't the last flying attempt of the Lilienthal brothers. For the next seventeen years the boys spent every penny they had on gliders. Then Gustav seems to have lost interest. Otto went on experimenting by himself.

Otto and Gustav Lilienthal were born in Pomerania, a former province of Germany. Otto was born May 24, 1848, Gustav a year later. Their early attempts to make gliders with flapping wings were all failures. But, after Otto abandoned that idea and turned to fixed-wing gliders, he began making important contributions to flight. He is acknowledged as one of the greatest of the early pioneers in gliding.

Lilienthal believed that the only way to learn to fly was to do what the birds did—practice in the air. A pilot could only estimate how a craft would react to air currents until he flew it and found out. In 1891, Lilienthal built the first glider that got off the ground. It was made with a framework of tough willow rods and was covered with cotton twill shirting. The cotton was coated with a solution to make it as airtight as possible.

Otto Lilienthal made over two hundred glider flights in sixteen separate glider types to test his theories. His study of birds led him to build his glider wings with a curved upper surface. He was one of the first persons to understand that this shape would provide lift.

We are fortunate in having a firsthand account of Otto Lilienthal flying a glider when he was at the peak of his career. Although Lilienthal's work received little notice in Europe, his daring exploits captured the imagination of people in the United States. Recent improvements had been made in the wire services and in photography. Articles and photographs could be sent across the Atlantic in minutes, to appear in magazines and newspapers here. Startling pictures of a man soaring in the air intrigued Americans. The *Boston Transcript* sent a reporter, Robert W. Wood, to Berlin to interview Otto Lilienthal. Mr. Wood sent back an enthusiastic account of one of Lilienthal's flights, complete with photographs.

The machine that Otto Lilienthal flew for Mr. Wood on August 2, 1896, was a biplane. Like all his gliders, this one was clearly patterned after a bird. While Robert Wood set up his camera, the glider was carried to the crest of a hill. Mr. Lilienthal crawled under it, put his arms through some cuffs, and grasped a bar near the forward edge of the wing. He stood there for a moment as the wind freshened. Then he ran about three steps down the hill and was flying. He soared about 50 feet over the head of the astonished Mr. Wood.

During that afternoon, Lilienthal made ten different flights. The reporter was overcome with admiration for the wild fearlessness of this flying man supported by his huge white wings. At last Robert Wood asked if he could make a flight. Lilienthal readily agreed. After Wood had been helped into the machine, he was almost ready to back out.

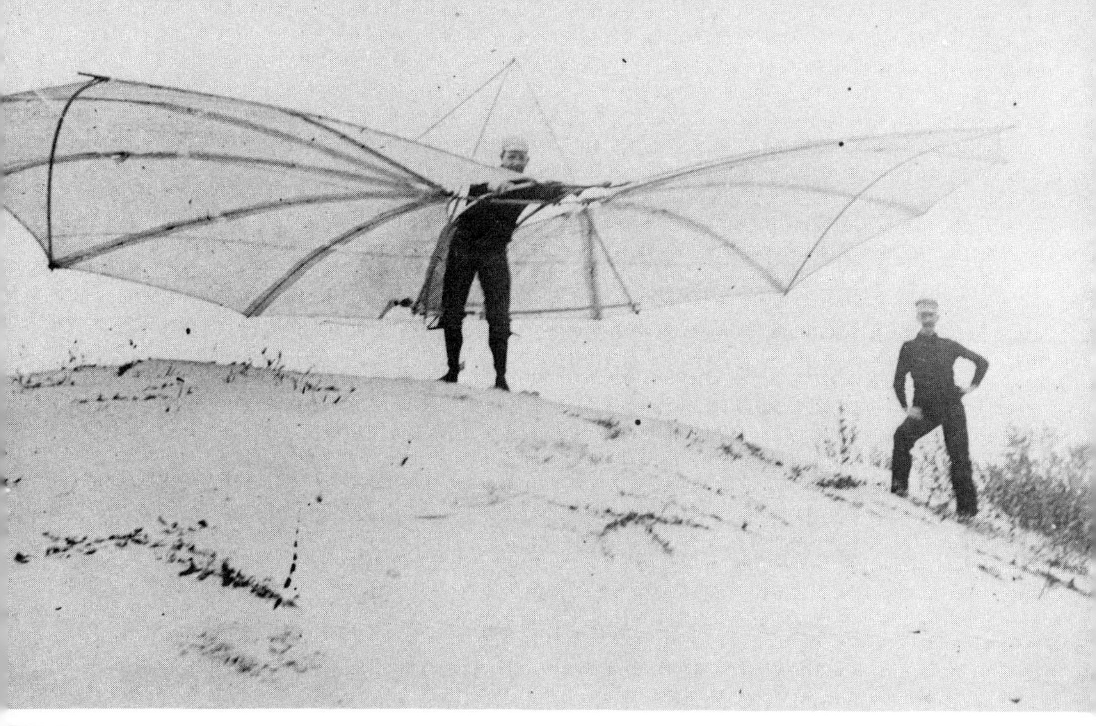

A. M. Herring about to fly a Lilienthal glider

He found it so difficult to balance the heavy wings that he felt utterly helpless. But when Lilienthal told him to run downhill, he began to stagger forward. To his surprise he found that the huge wings became lighter with each step he took. Suddenly he realized that his feet were no longer touching the ground. Mr. Wood's flight wasn't very long, but he sent an enthusiastic account back to Boston.

After Mr. Wood's visit with Mr. Lilienthal, he planned to go back for a follow-up interview. On the following Sunday, Otto Lilienthal was again out flying—this time a monoplane. On one of his flights he stalled and fell 50 feet to the ground, breaking his spine. The daring airman died the next day in a Berlin hospital at the age of forty-eight. His last words were, "This is the price of progress."

On all of Lilienthal's gliders, the pilot hung between the wings. The glider was controlled by the movement of the pilot's torso and legs. This is the way hang glider pilots control their machines today. Although Lilienthal's gliders were a forerunner of today's hang gliders, they also contributed to the development of both the glider and the airplane. Lilienthal saw the hang glider as a necessary intermediate step toward the development of powered flight. He looked at the problems of flight as a steady process of evolution. First would come the simple hang glider, then a more sophisticated glider, then a glider with an engine—an airplane.

Lilienthal sold one of his gliders to William Randolph Hearst, the newspaperman. It can now be seen in the Smithsonian Institution. He sold plans of other gliders to flying enthusiasts in the United States. A. M. Herring built and flew several Lilienthal hang gliders. Lilienthal's feats aroused great enthusiasm in the United States and led to the founding of the first glider club in America. He is considered the father of hang gliding.

JOHN JOSEPH MONTGOMERY

John Joseph Montgomery was a controversial figure in the history of gliding. Once he visited Octave Chanute, who, at that time, was writing his book about flying machines. Montgomery gave Chanute an account of his gliding flights for the book. But afterward he changed his stories many times. With each account his flights became longer and higher.

Montgomery was born in California in 1858. He too became interested in the flight of birds while he was still a child. About 1880 he began to design and build hang gliders that could carry a person. His first designs, all based on birds, were failures. In 1884, though, he built a successful fixed-wing glider with a 20-foot wingspan. The pilot rode in a seat suspended under the frame.

John Montgomery found the ideal place to fly this monoplane glider at Otay Mesa, south of San Diego. On the morning of his test flight, a steady sea breeze made for ideal flying conditions. John sat in the seat and grasped the two central bars of the frame. He gave a slight jump and found himself skimming down the slope with his feet off the ground. On his first flight, as he later told Chanute, he covered about one hundred feet. On his next try, the glider crashed.

Montgomery often had other men fly his gliders. One of his stunts was to use a hot-air balloon to lift the glider high in the air. Daniel Maloney, a pilot for Montgomery, made some spectacular flights by launching the glider from beneath a balloon. He would drop 3,000 to 4,000 feet while

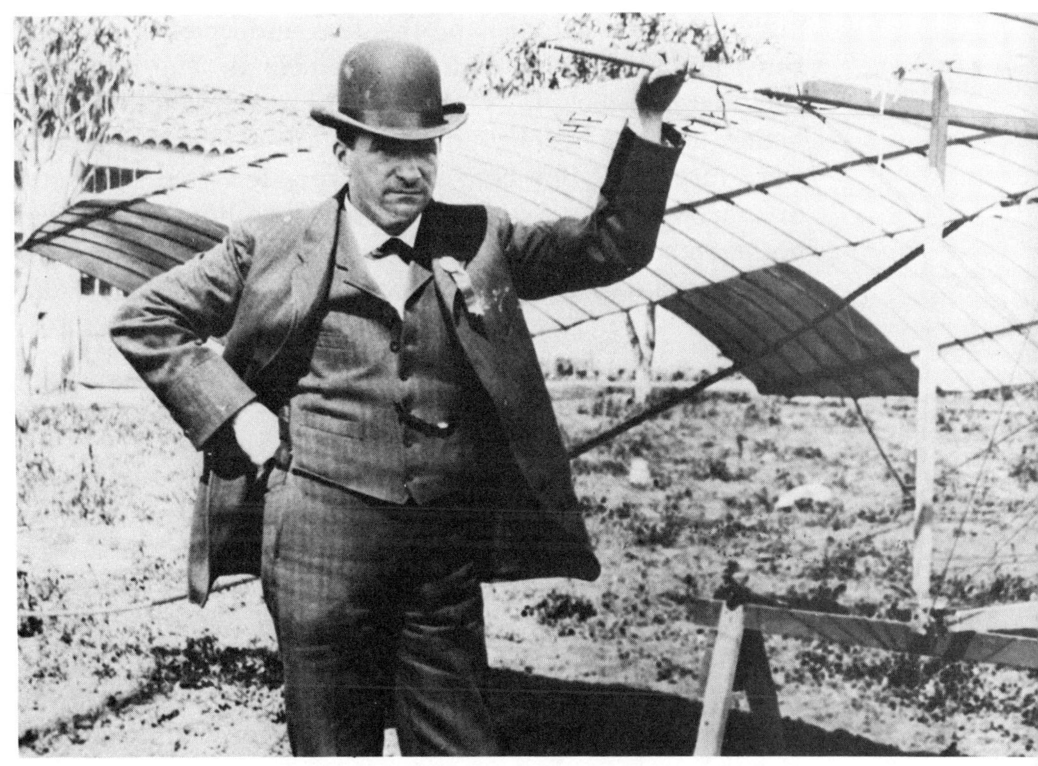

John Montgomery poses with his 1905 glider

swooping, soaring, and gliding. Unfortunately Maloney was killed on one of these flights. Later, Montgomery too fell to his death while flying one of his gliders.

Cayley, Lilienthal, and Montgomery were all convinced that a curved upper surface on the wing provided lift. But, unaccountably, this fact was forgotten and rediscovered several times.

HANG GLIDERS ARE FORGOTTEN

After the Wright brothers put an engine in a glider and flew, the age of powered flight began. People lost interest in gliders. But gradually sailplanes made a comeback. Flying enthusiasts enjoyed the freedom and quiet of soaring. But sailplanes soon became sophisticated. The pilot was enclosed in a cockpit. As designs improved, sailplanes flew higher and faster. The slower and lower forms of gliding were forgotten. But here and there a few free souls still dreamed of really flying like a bird—but how? There was no machine to fly with. Engineers knew more about flying at supersonic speeds than about flying at 25 miles per hour.

FRANCIS M. ROGALLO

Sixty years after hang gliders were forgotten, flying like a bird was to make a comeback. It all started with Francis Rogallo, an aeronautical engineer with Langley Research Center in Hampton, Virginia. In 1936 he was testing wings in a wind tunnel. He was trying to find out which shape provided the most lift. Rogallo began to wonder if cloth, attached to a frame, wouldn't billow out in flight into the same shape and provide the same lift as the wings he was testing.

Rogallo built a triangular-shaped kite frame and covered

it loosely with cloth. His wife, Gertrude, joined him in the experiments. In the wind tunnel the cloth billowed into a curved surface. This should provide the same lift as a solid wing. After more tests, the wing was patented in 1951.

But what use was a cloth wing? No one seemed to know. Francis Rogallo later went to work for the National Aeronautics and Space Administration (NASA). He offered them his new wing if they could find a use for it. Experiments were made. NASA was interested in using the wing as a sort of parachute to ferry space vehicles back to earth. The Army experimented with it. They found that a jeep could glide safely to earth attached to a Rogallo wing. When attached to an 8-ton load, a helicopter could tow it without loss of power. This wing had the advantage of being maneuverable. It offered forward movement as well as lift. But these ideas never got beyond the experimental stage. NASA couldn't figure out a use for the wing—so it was forgotten. Like many other great ideas, it would have been lost forever—except for one thing. NASA published a description of the Rogallo wing and sent it out to interested people.

Around the world there were still people who dreamed of flying in a simple, uncomplicated way. Fortunately a few of them read NASA's report on the Rogallo wing.

BARRY HILL PALMER

Barry Hill Palmer of California read NASA's article and built a Rogallo wing. He found he could run and take off on the sand dunes beside the Pacific Ocean. A few short flights were made with this first wing. Palmer usually gets the credit for being the first person to hang glide in modern times.

THOMAS PURCELL

Across the United States on the Atlantic Coast, another flying enthusiast read NASA's article. This was Thomas Purcell of North Carolina. He built a Rogallo wing and tried it while being towed by a motorboat. Purcell is given credit for being the first person to hang glide with a tow. But these two experiments with the Rogallo wing received little publicity. It remained for two Australians to popularize hang gliding in the United States.

WILLIAM BENNETT AND WILLIAM MOYES

Let's see what was going on at 7,316-foot-high Mt. Kosciusko one winter day in August. The low afternoon sun had given the snow on Mt. Kosciusko a rosy cast. The pink-tinted ski slope stretched down the flank of Australia's highest mountain. It was late in the day and most of the skiers had gone, when two men on skis, one with some sort of large kite, appeared at the top of the ski slope.

Then, as the amazed skiers watched, the man with the kite launched himself down the ski slope. He was followed by the other man on skis. Every now and then the man with the kite rose from the snow and made a short glide before returning to the ski slope. After skiing over a higher rise, the skier and kite continued to soar. Then one wing shot up into the air and the flying skier took a dive into a snowbank.

The friend who had accompanied the winged skier now sideslipped down to him. The friend unfastened the broken wings and helped the man to his feet. The deep snow on Mt. Kosciusko had cushioned the fall.

William Bennett and William Moyes gathered up the broken wings and headed for the parking lot. They were going to spend the night with a friend in New South Wales. As they drove to his house, they talked about their experiments. In 1956 the two friends had begun to design and build wing-shaped kites. Their kites featured cloth stretched tightly over a frame. They had tried towing a water-skier, wearing this kite, behind a powerboat. The kite would lift a person out of the water. But in the air the kite was erratic. When the forward motion stopped, the wing dived into the water. If the men hadn't done their flying over water or snow, they would long ago have been killed.

Their friend in New South Wales was excited when the two Bills arrived. He had been following their experiments.

"How did it go today?" he asked. He was greeted by gloomy looks and shaking heads. "Well, have I got something for you two to see. I think it may be the answer to your problem."

What the friend had to show Bill Bennett and Bill Moyes was NASA's report on the Rogallo wing. After they read the article, many things became clear to the two inventors. Because the top surface of their kite was flat, it created no lift. What they had was a kite. It only generated lift while it was being towed or was fastened to someone traveling at high speed. But if there was slack in the cloth covering their wing, as described in the NASA report, their wing should have lift.

Bennett and Moyes immediately went to work on a kite somewhat like the Rogallo wing. They towed this new wing behind a powerboat with excellent success. But they still thought of it as a kite that must be towed. One day the towrope broke while Bennett was at a considerable height. With their old kite, this would have been a disaster. But the wing continued to soar before finally gliding gently down to earth. The loose cloth had billowed out in flight and provided stability and lift. Soon both Moyes and Bennett were soaring. They became accomplished hang glider pilots.

Bill Bennett and Bill Moyes decided to take their new glider to the United States. Here their stunts attracted wide attention. Bill Bennett, pulled by a motorboat, soared over San Francisco Bay and under the Golden Gate Bridge. Finally he cut himself loose and landed on Alcatraz Island.

Later the two men went to New York City. Here Bill Bennett was towed around the Statue of Liberty. Then he cut himself loose and spiraled slowly to the ground.

The men began to launch themselves from high places instead of being towed. Bennett jumped from a mountain near Death Valley, California. He soared until finally landing in Death Valley, over a mile below his starting point. Moyes jumped off the rim of the Grand Canyon, soaring and gliding to the canyon floor far below.

All the newspapers published photographs and articles about the gliding stunts of these two Australians. Many people who dreamed of someday flying like a bird realized that that day was here. Bill Bennett and Bill Moyes, more than anyone else, popularized hang gliding. The sport first caught on in California. Quickly it spread all over the West Coast, then to the rest of the United States. Within a few years people all over the world were hang gliding.

Most hang gliders today use the Rogallo wing. It is the safest and easiest wing to fly. Unfortunately for Francis Rogallo, his patent expired in 1968. He collects nothing from those who manufacture and sell Rogallo wings. This invention has brought him fame but not fortune.

4. FLYING LIKE A BIRD

ARE HANG GLIDER PILOTS DAREDEVILS?

It was July in Yosemite National Park. Tourists crowded the valley floor. Some of them watched the falls cascading to the valley below. Some admired Half Dome or El Capitan lit by the midday sun. Some swam or sunbathed on the sandy beaches of Merced River. The more active played tennis or bicycled. Then, as if by magic, all activity ceased. Automobile brakes screeched and cars blocked valley roads. No one ran after the bouncing tennis balls. They came to rest unnoticed. The bicyclists stopped beside the road and braced themselves on one leg. The swimmers stood in the shallow water. On all the trails the hikers no longer admired the natural beauty of the valley. Had the wicked witch cast a spell again? No, this sudden freezing of all the visitors in Yosemite Valley happens quite often. Now take a good look at all those motionless people. Their heads are all tipped back. All are gazing up at Glacier Point. What are they watching?

Glacier Point is an outcropping of rock on a cliff towering 3,000 feet above Yosemite Valley. When the sun has warmed the valley floor, warm air rises up past Glacier Point. A paved road leading to this point makes it ideal for hang gliders. But whenever little black figures begin to spiral high above the valley, all traffic stops. Those who have never seen this sight before think, at first, that they are watching some new species of gigantic bird. But, as the specks circle lower, the human bodies under the wings are visible.

If you could listen to the watching people, you would hear something like this:

"Look at those daredevils."

"I wouldn't do that for a million dollars."

"They must be tired of living."

"I hope his insurance is paid up."

Is hang gliding that dangerous? Are the pilots really daredevils? Well, hang gliding is not, in itself, dangerous. But when you are 3,000 feet up and hanging from an aluminum frame and cloth wings, there is no place for carelessness. If the pilot is careful, the sport can be enjoyed in relative safety. The urge to show off is the one thing that causes the most accidents. The old saying about flying is also true for hang gliding. "There are old pilots and there are bold pilots. But there are no old, bold pilots."

Another good adage for beginning hang glider pilots is, "Don't fly higher than you are willing to fall." The beginner often underestimates the dangers of the sport. Experienced pilots make it look so easy. The novice should only undertake hang gliding with good equipment and under the supervision of a U.S. Hang Gliding Association (USHGA) instructor. He or she should purchase the first wing from a reputable dealer, not try to build it. Only an expert knows enough about aerodynamics to build a wing. All equipment, including the harness, should be checked before each flight.

Safety equipment is necessary. You will see photographs of hang gliders with the pilot's hair blowing in the breeze. That may feel good, but unless you are very lucky, you will make only a few flights that way. A crash helmet should be worn at all times. Many pilots are alive today because they were wearing a crash helmet during a rough landing. A heavy jacket, jeans, gloves, and kneepads help prevent nasty scrapes. Flotation gear is necessary if there is any chance that you might land in water. While learning, you should fly only when the wind is blowing from zero to fifteen miles per hour. Wind speed should be checked with a wind meter —this is not the time or the place to play guessing games.

Care is always necessary. The unexpected can happen and sometimes it does. Equipment failure or a rapid change in weather conditions are two ever-present dangers. At times even experienced hang glider pilots have serious accidents.

Do you remember Bill Bennett and Bill Moyes from Australia? In the spring of 1970, Bill Moyes was doing a show in Sydney, Australia. A car was towing his kite so he could gain altitude. The car went too fast and the kite came apart in the air. Bill Moyes fell several hundred feet onto a parked car. He received serious injuries, including a fractured pelvis. In June 1971, Bill Bennett misjudged a landing. He crashed into a fence and received several crushed vertebrae.

Hang gliding can be dangerous. It requires care if you are to do it safely. And even care does not always prevent an accident. Let's take a closer look at hang gliders.

WHAT IS A HANG GLIDER?

Before we talk more about the hang glider, let's get a few terms straightened out. What is a hang glider? Very simply, it is a glider from which the pilot hangs. This does not mean that the pilot hangs on with the hands or arms. He or she is suspended below a wing on a swing seat or in a harness and rides in a sitting or prone position. Some hang gliders have wings like a monoplane or a biplane sailplane. But if the pilot's legs provide the energy for launching and land-

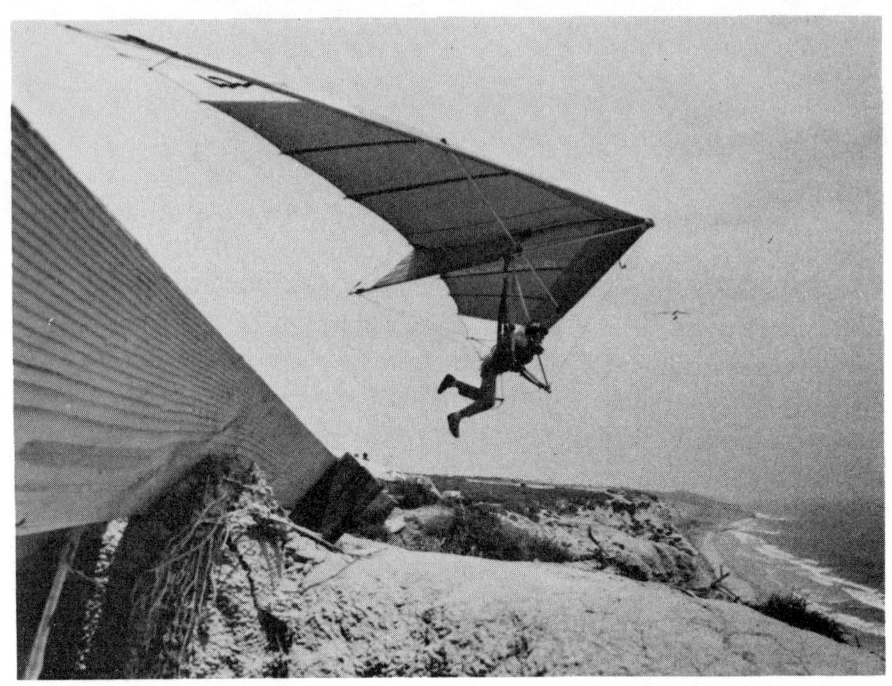

Taking off from a cliff with a Rogallo wing

ing, the craft is officially a hang glider.

Ninety percent of the hang gliders flown today are based on the Rogallo design. The aluminum tubing frame is fashioned in the shape of a giant A. The keel boom runs from the leading edge, the point of the A, straight back. Dacron cloth is stretched loosely over this frame. In flight, the cloth fills with air to billow out and produce lift. The entire machine only weighs from thirty to fifty pounds and can easily be folded up and transported on top of a car.

The Rogallo wing is the easiest hang glider to fly, launch, and transport. The beginner should stick with it. Rigid-wing gliders, both monoplane and biplane, are being built today that have a better overall performance than the Rogallo wing. But since they are trickier to fly, they should be flown only by experienced pilots. They also require the assistance of several people on takeoff.

In flight the Rogallo wing obeys Bernoulli's principle,

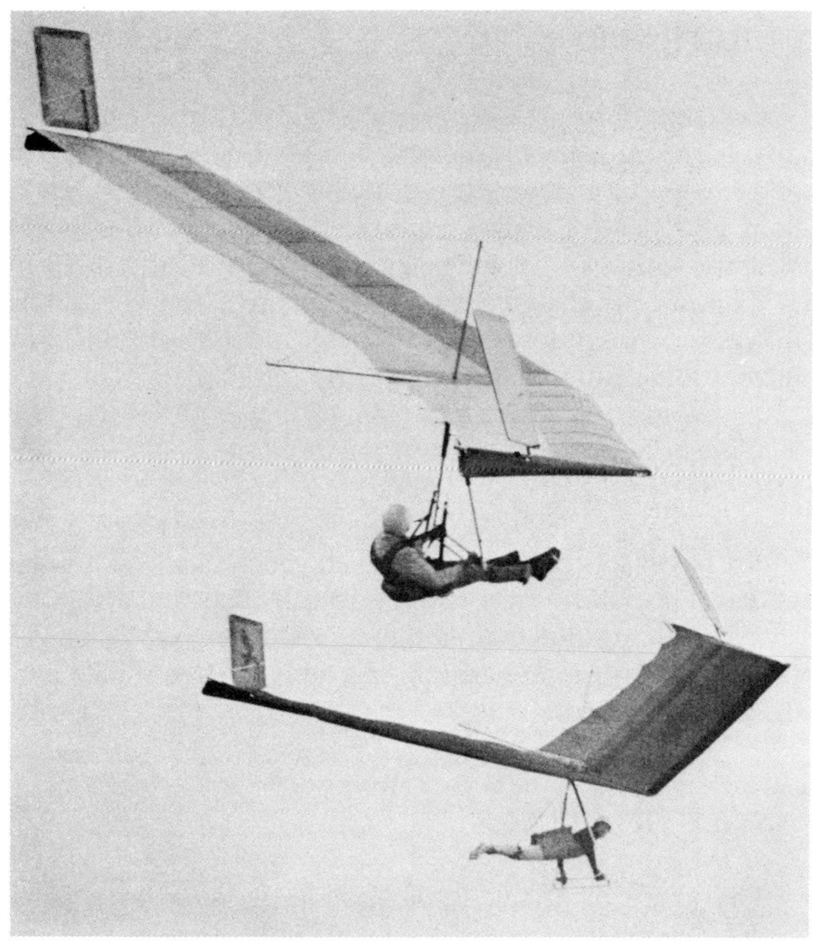

Rigid-wing hang gliders are more difficult to fly

just as do all wings. The curved upper surface provides lift.
But because the hang glider and the pilot are heavier than
air, they begin to go down the minute the pilot steps off a
cliff. The lift provided by the shape of the wing keeps the
pilot from falling straight down. The pilot glides forward,
always descending, until reaching the ground or encounter-
ing an updraft of air.

GLIDE RATIO

Different hang gliders descend at different rates of speed, just as do sailplanes. The sinking speed, or glide ratio, is determined by the weight and shape of the wings. Rogallo hang gliders have a glide ratio of about 4 to 1. Monoplane designs, with a wider wingspan, often have a ratio of 10 to 1. This means that for every four or five feet the glider moves forward, it loses one foot in altitude. Most sailplanes have a glide ratio of at least 26 to 1.

DRAG

Air passing over the glider and the pilot's body slows the glider. This is known as drag. Drag increases the sinking speed of a hang glider; streamlining reduces drag. When the pilot flies in a prone position, the body is streamlined and drag is decreased.

ANGLE OF ATTACK

The angle of attack is of vital importance to a hang glider. This is the angle at which the leading or forward edge of the wing meets the air as it moves through it. The

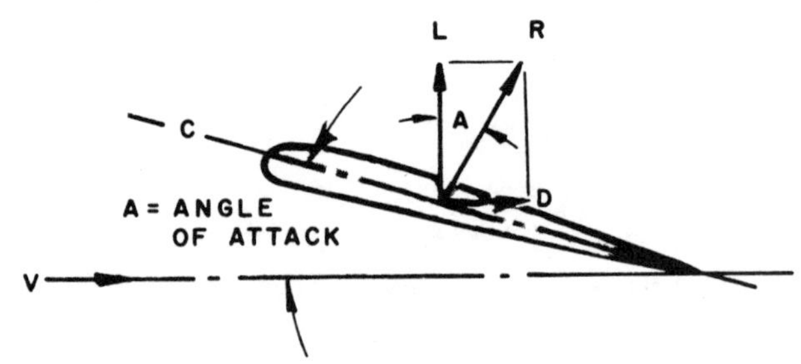

The angle of attack controls glider lift

leading edge of the wing is normally slightly elevated during flight. When the angle of attack is increased, air moves over the wing more rapidly and additional lift is produced. But, at the same time, more of the underside of the wing is exposed and drag is increased. If the angle of the wing is increased higher than fifty degrees, drag becomes stronger than lift. When the wing no longer produces lift, the machine goes into a stall. Unless prompt action is taken, the glider falls to the ground.

If the leading edge of the wing is dipped lower than a 15-degree angle, the puffed-out cloth of the wing collapses. The pilot loses lift and falls. This is known as a flag fall, because the pilot hears the wing flapping like a flag in a breeze. The leading edge of the wing must be brought up quickly to prevent disaster.

SOARING

Hang gliders use updrafts of warm air to gain altitude just as do sailplanes. In the section on gliders, we discussed the different types of updrafts used by sailplane pilots— ridge lifts, thermals, and mountain or lee waves. All of these are also used by hang glider pilots. But you will find most of these enthusiasts soaring over ridge lifts. Hang gliding first gained popularity when pilots discovered the ridge lifts over the sea cliffs on the Southern California coast. What causes these predictable updrafts of air over sea cliffs? During the day, the sun heats the land in certain places and warm air begins to rise. Sea cliffs, since they are usually composed of exposed rock and dirt, heat up faster than vegetation. The colder air over the water moves in to replace the rising warm air. This creates a steady onshore wind that is ideal for hang gliding. Toward the end of the day, the land cools off and the wind becomes weak. Then the hang glider enthusiasts fold their wings and head for

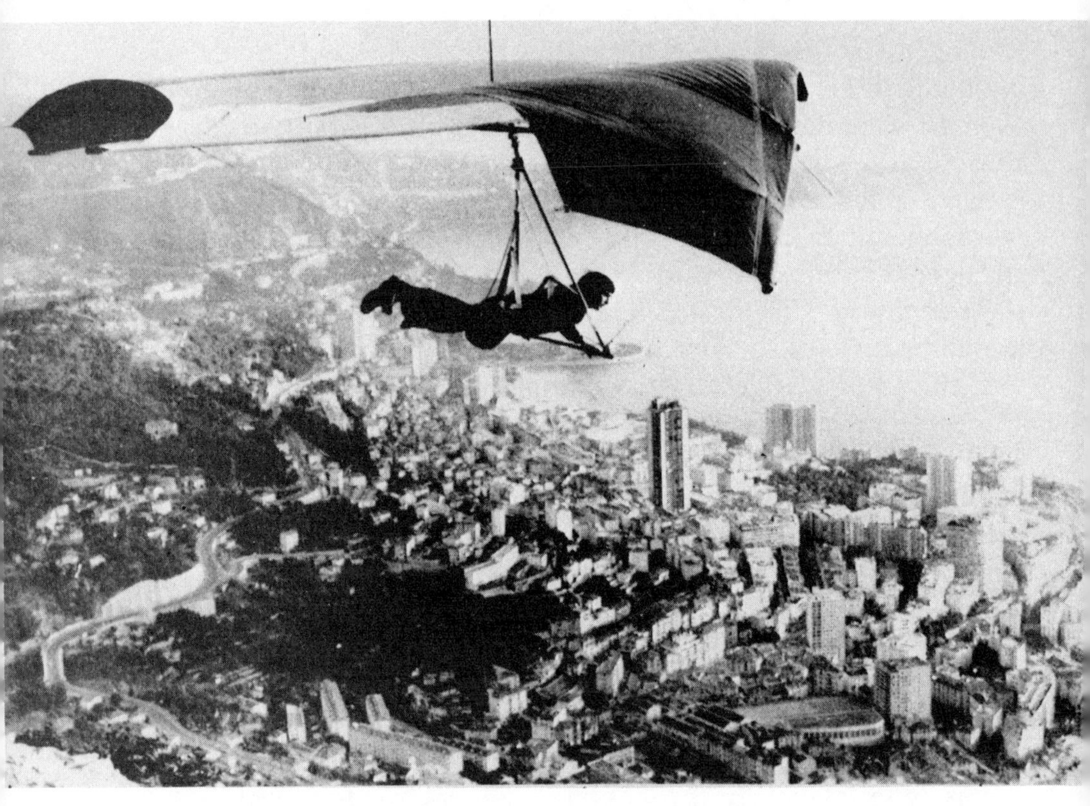

Hang glider utilizing a ridge lift over Monaco

home. But as soon as the land warms up the next day, the breeze returns.

A hang glider can fly back and forth in a ridge lift. These same updrafts also occur near mountains. You will often find hang gliders clustered on a mountain cliff that drops steeply to a valley below. This sport often requires the pilot to clamber up a steep slope carrying the wing. For that reason, hang glider pilots are usually young people in excellent physical condition.

Vast areas of the United States are not provided with sea cliffs or mountains that produce ridge lifts. There are miles and miles of flat country with never a hill. But there are many thermals in flat land. As we found out in the section

58

on sailplanes, thermals occur whenever the land is heated unevenly. But in order to take advantage of a thermal, the hang glider must start from a height. In flat country, the only way to achieve the needed altitude is with a tow. Motorboats can be used to tow a hang glider on water skis. When snow is on the ground, a car or snowmobile can be used to tow a hang glider on snow skis. Skiers can also launch themselves by skiing downhill.

Towing can be tricky. Only an expert should try it. A Rogallo wing cannot be used, as it won't stand the stress of the tow. Only rigid hang gliders, which are harder to handle, can be used.

HOW TO FLY A HANG GLIDER

The Rogallo wing has a rigid control bar fastened to the frame. The pilot rides suspended in a harness. The pilot uses this control bar to push forward or backward. When the pilot pulls forward, the nose of the glider tips down. The glider gains speed and loses altitude. When the pilot pushes backward, the tail tips down. The glider gains lift but loses speed.

Now how about turning? The pilot does that by changing the center of gravity. Every object, or combination of objects, has a center of gravity. You can balance a long pole on your finger if you find the center of gravity. The pilot and hang glider together have a center of gravity. When the pilot hangs in a normal flying position, the wings are level. When the pilot moves the body to one side, the glider tilts and turns. A hang glider pilot turns by moving the body in the desired direction.

Taking off is easier than landing. The pilot can wait until conditions are right. If there isn't much wind, the hang glider pilot runs down a slope to create enough airflow over the wing surface to generate lift. This is the way a beginner

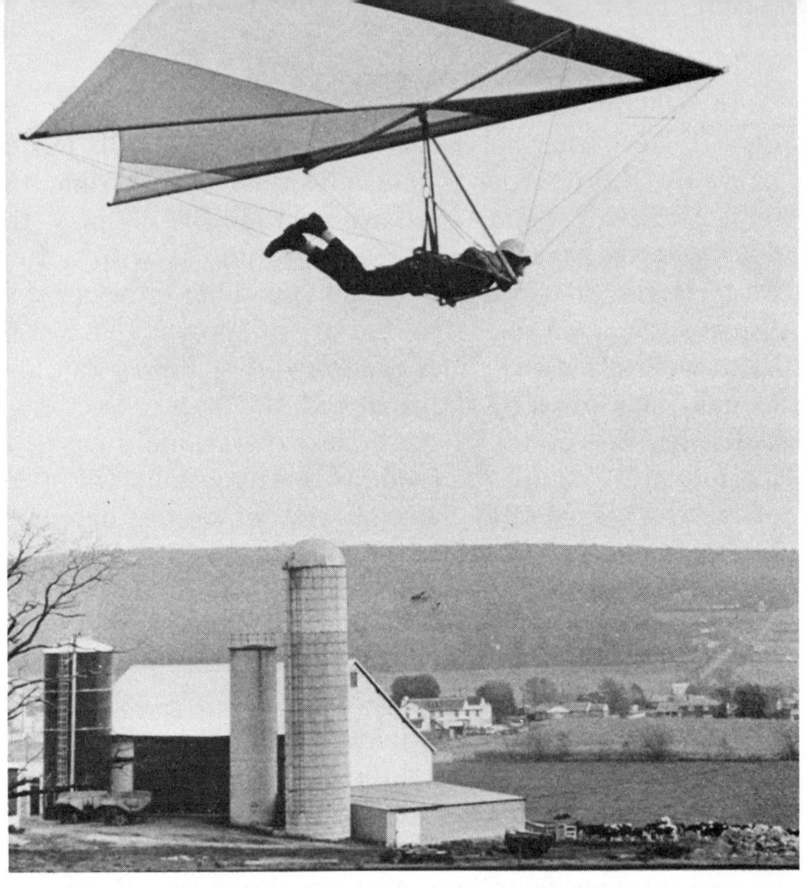

A prone position decreases drag

should learn how to take off. But a timid takeoff won't work. You must run as fast as possible and launch yourself forcefully. Speed is necessary to get airborne. A halfhearted effort will result in a stall and crash.

If there is a brisk wind and a high place to take off from, the expert pilot can just push off. Taking off on a slope would seem to be safer. But there is always the danger of a sudden gust of wind or too slow a speed producing a stall. Taking off from a cliff is safer. The pilot has altitude from the start. In hang gliding, altitude means safety.

Landing is much more difficult. You must make judgments instantly. Hesitation can be fatal. To avoid a fall, the wing must maintain lift until your feet touch ground. You

60

will be pulled up if the wing still continues to lift. For a perfect landing, the glider should be put into a stall the moment your feet touch the ground. Then start running. Otherwise the forward momentum of the glider will pull you off your feet.

GETTING INTO HANG GLIDING

If you want more information about hang gliding, write to the U.S. Hang Gliding Association, Box 66306, Los Angeles, California 90066. They will send you information about clubs, certified dealers, and flight schools in your area. With this information you can go to the places where hang glider pilots meet and talk to them and watch them fly. But don't try the sport on your own. Get your instruction from a qualified instructor. There are schools that teach hang gliding and basic flight theory. They will also advise you about the equipment suitable for beginners. The novice becomes a better pilot, learns faster, and lives longer if instruction is taken at a hang gliding flight school.

PART THREE / *PARACHUTING*

5. FROM PARASOLS TO PARACHUTES

IT ALL BEGAN IN CHINA

Emperor Shih Huang Ti strolled along the newly completed Great Wall. Proudly he gazed at the fortification, which stretched as far as he could see. It climbed mountains and dipped into valleys until it finally disappeared behind a distant hill. At last China had a strong defense against its warlike neighbors to the north.

A huge festival would be held at the time of the next full moon to celebrate the completion of this project. There would be dancers, jugglers, acrobats, and musicians. The emperor wanted to do something himself—but what?

A few weeks later the full moon shone on a colorful sight. Paper lanterns glowed along both sides of the Great Wall. Firecrackers popped and skyrockets flowered. Troops of performers entertained the crowds.

Then the boom of drums and the clash of gongs announced the arrival of the emperor. Before him marched his musicians and the royal guard. His family and ministers followed at a respectful distance. Shih Huang Ti, the mighty conqueror, was feared by all his subjects. But on this occasion he radiated goodwill. In his purple robe embroidered with gold threads, he advanced slowly along the wall, smiling at everyone. The people bowed low as their lord strode past them.

The emperor, it had been announced, would perform a daring feat at the celebration. Everyone followed the procession, eager to see what it would be. At a wider spot, overlooking the valley, the emperor stopped and raised his hand. Instantly the crowds ceased their shoving and chattering.

The emperor thanked his people for their years of work on the wall. "Now," he said, "you will be safe from the fierce barbarians to the north." Then he added, "Many of you have performed stunts to entertain others on this great occasion. Your emperor wishes to do something too. Tonight I am going to perform a feat never before accomplished. I will jump from the Great Wall."

A murmur arose from the crowds. The wall was 25 feet high. But, at this place, it was built on the side of the hill and was 100 feet above the ground. Several of the ministers came forward to try to persuade the emperor not to jump. But he waved them all aside and strode to the edge of the wall. There he climbed onto the parapet and motioned to one of his attendants. The man came forward and handed a huge parasol to the emperor.

People ran to the edge of the wall to watch. Down below, the emperor had stationed guards with flares. Now he opened the huge parasol. The wind tugged at it, making it difficult to hold. The emperor waved at the crowds, grasped the handle of the parasol and jumped. The wind caught the parasol and, for a time, the ruler was higher than the wall. His robe billowed out in the breeze. Then the parasol and the emperor floated gradually down to earth. A tremendous roar went up from the people massed on the wall.

Did the Chinese emperor Shih Huang Ti really make a parasol jump over two thousand years ago? That we shall never know. Legends are a mixture of fact and fiction that are impossible to separate centuries later. But an old Chinese legend says Emperor Shih safely made several such

64

jumps from the Great Wall.

The Chinese have many stories about people jumping from high places while holding on to something to trap air and slow the fall. For that reason it is generally believed that the Chinese were the first to use a parachute. An ancient legend credits Emperor Shun (2258-2208 B.C.) with being the first person to use a parachute. But we have no idea of the kind of parachute used.

The Chinese have another story about a jump from a high place. Long ago in Pingting, Li-ying, a poor Chinese farmer, fell in love with Po-bok, the daughter of a wealthy landlord. When Po-bok was only six years old, the father had betrothed her to an old but wealthy merchant. Li-ying was forbidden to see Po-bok. But several days each month the father went away to collect rents from his tenants. While her father was away, Po-bok sent word to Li-ying to meet her in the garden.

One evening the young lovers walked and talked among the flowers. Suddenly the garden gate opened and there was the girl's father. He let out a roar of rage when he saw Li-ying and Po-bok together. Drawing his broad sword, he advanced on the young man. Li-ying was terrified. Looking for a way to escape, he ran into the house and up a flight of stairs. The father ran after him, slashing with his sword and yelling. Po-bok ran after her father, pleading for her lover's life.

Li-ying ran up another flight of stairs. He opened a trapdoor and climbed out onto the roof. But the father was right behind him. Li-ying was trapped. With raised sword the angry father advanced on the young man. Li-ying had come to see Po-bok directly from work in the fields and still wore his working clothes. In desperation he took off his large, circular coolie's hat. Then, holding the hat by each side, he jumped from the roof.

The angry father ran to the edge of the roof and looked down. He expected to see the young man lying dead below.

But the hat had trapped enough air to break Li-ying's fall. Quickly the young man jumped to his feet, vaulted over the garden wall, and disappeared into the night.

Whether or not this legend is true, we have no way of knowing. But we do know that Oriental actors and acrobats commonly used large parasols in their stunts. An acrobat would leap from a high place onto the stage while holding on to the handle of a parasol. Simon de la Loubère was the French Ambassador to Siam in the 1680s. He wrote about a tumbler who amused the King of Siam by leaping from a high platform with two umbrellas fastened to his girdle. Sometimes the wind carried him into a tree; sometimes onto the roof; sometimes into the river. The king so enjoyed this stunt that he had the tumbler come live in the palace and made him a great lord.

The idea for the parachute undoubtedly came from the parasol or umbrella. Anyone who has tried to hold on to an umbrella in a high wind knows umbrellas can trap a great quantity of air. Such an experience may have given someone, living hundreds of years ago, the idea of using one as a parachute.

LEONARDO DA VINCI

Europeans had little contact with the Orient until the eighteenth century. Some of the things invented by the Chinese many centuries ago were later reinvented by Europeans. Although we think of Leonardo da Vinci as an artist, he was also an inventor. He was interested in all sorts of devices. You will remember that he drew plans for a flying machine. Around 1480 he also drew plans for a parachute. He called it a tent roof. Leonardo's design for a glider could not have flown. But the design for the parachute was sound. Leonardo da Vinci's description of his parachute reads: "If a man has a tent roof of caulked linen twelve braccia broad

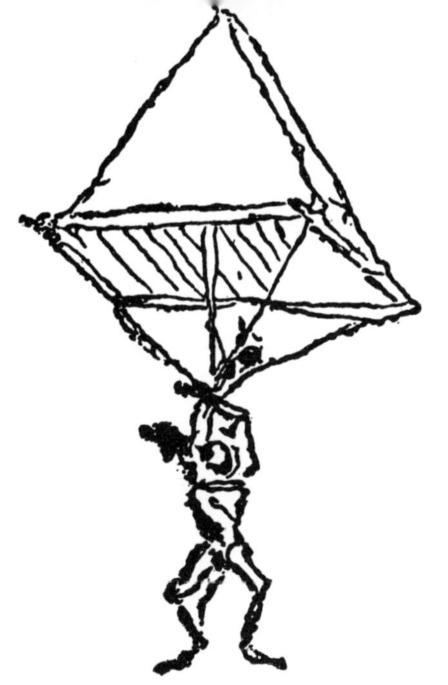

and twelve braccia high, he will be able to let himself fall from a great height without danger to himself."

A braccio is approximately one yard. So Leonardo's parachute would have been about 36 feet wide and 36 feet from base to apex. Linen, painted with something to make it airtight, was to be stretched over a wooden frame. A pole would be fastened to the top of the parachute and extend below it. The parachutist would hang from this pole and hold on to a cord from each corner.

There is no record that anyone ever built and used Leonardo's parachute. But if lightweight wood were used, the parachute should support the weight of a man in the air.

After Leonardo's death in 1519, his sketches were stored away. No one seemed to realize their importance. It wasn't until the end of the nineteenth century that a selection of his aeronautical sketches, including the one of a parachute, were published. So again the parachute was invented and forgotten.

In 1595, Fausto Veranzio of Venice published a book called *New Machines*. For the first time, an engraving of a parachute appeared. It was labeled *Homo volans,* or flying man. The sketch showed a man jumping from a tower with a square parachute. Veranzio evidently understood drag. He stated that the size of the frame should vary according to the weight of the man. Generally, a larger canopy produces more drag and so can sustain a greater weight.

In 1617, Veranzio built the parachute shown in the sketch. It consisted of a wooden frame covered with canvas. With this parachute he planned on jumping from a tower in St. Mark's Square, Venice. For some reason this jump was never made.

JOSEPH MONTGOLFIER

Joseph and Étienne Montgolfier are famous as the inventors of the hot-air balloon. But five years before he became interested in ballooning, Joseph was experimenting with parachutes. Between 1777 and 1779 he dropped several sheep from a high tower in Annonay, France. Each one survived the fall fastened to a 7-foot parachute that looked something like a big parasol. Joseph Montgolfier also tried parachuting. He made a successful jump from a housetop in Annonay.

SÉBASTIEN LENORMAND

Sébastien Lenormand was a professor of physics and chemistry at Montpellier, France. He seems an unlikely person to risk his life by jumping off a tower. But that is just what he did. He wanted to test his theory that a large canopy would provide enough resistance to air to enable a body to descend safely to earth. He built a cone-shaped parachute of oiled silk 14 feet in diameter. On December 26, 1783, he donned this contraption and stepped off the tower of the Montpellier Observatory. Although he came down rather hard, he was unharmed. Later, Professor Lenormand made a safe jump from the upper story of a house. He believed his parachute could be used as a safety device for escape from the upper floors of burning buildings.

Sébastien Lenormand is credited with coining the word "parachute." It is derived from the Italian verb *parare,* meaning to protect, and the French noun *chute,* meaning fall.

PARACHUTING FROM BALLOONS

In a few years after the first balloon flight in 1783, balloons were all the rage. Every festival or fair had a balloon ascension. But sometimes a strong wind caught the balloon and carried it away. Sometimes the bag burst or caught fire. Sometimes a balloon was blown out to sea. These early balloonists needed a safe way to return to earth when necessary. Parachutes seemed to be the answer. The early balloonists were also the early parachutists.

The early parachutes didn't look like the ones in use today. They consisted of a square or circular framework covered with cloth, and were not folded up. The parachute was suspended underneath the balloon's basket to be cut loose when needed. The parachutist rode either in the basket or on a trapeze fastened to the handle of the parachute. Tricks were often performed as the parachute floated back to earth.

Disasters were common in the days of early balloon ascensions and parachute descents. In London in August 1785, Stuart Arnold prepared for a balloon ascension. Underneath his balloon hung an open silk parachute. George Appleby was in the shallow basket tied to the parachute. Crowds of people were there to see him make a parachute jump from one mile up.

While the bag was being filled with hydrogen, Stuart Arnold's young son begged to be allowed to get into the basket. The father lifted him in, planning to put him out before the launching. Suddenly a gust of wind blew across the field and the balloon broke loose. It hit a railing and both Appleby and Arnold fell out. The frightened boy was carried up, up, up. Without the weight of the two men, the balloon rose faster and higher than planned. Hydrogen expands when altitude is increased. The gas in the balloon expanded until the bag burst.

As later balloonists discovered, when conditions are right the empty bag of a balloon can act like a parachute. In this case, the empty bag trapped enough air to slow the descent. The boy was thrown into the Thames River, while the balloon and parachute made a safe landing on the bank. The boy was fished out of the river unharmed.

JEAN-PIERRE BLANCHARD

Jean-Pierre Blanchard was a balloonist and a showman. In 1785, he began experimenting with dropping from his balloon animals attached to parachutes. On one occasion Blanchard dropped a terrified dog from a balloon. Then both the dog with the parachute and Blanchard in the balloon were swept up into the clouds. Blanchard could hear the dog yelping in the clouds, but never saw him again. Later Jean-Pierre made a silk parachute that could be folded up for easier transportation. He used it to release a dog, a cat, and a squirrel from an altitude of several thousand feet.

In 1801, Blanchard finally got up the courage to try a parachute jump himself. He broke his leg when landing. That was his first and last parachute jump.

GENERAL JEAN BOURNONVILLE

In 1793, General Jean Bournonville was sent by the newly formed French Republic to negotiate with the Prince of Saxe-Coburg. But the general and his aides were seized by the Austrians and placed in the fortress of Olmutz. Although imprisoned in a tower, General Bournonville was determined to escape. His only chance seemed to be flight by air. He jumped from a window holding on to the handle of a large umbrella. The general landed in a moat 40 feet below and broke his leg. Back he went to the tower.

ANDRÉ-JACQUES GARNERIN

Another Frenchman, André-Jacques Garnerin, was imprisoned by the Austrians in the same year. He had been sent by the French government to check on the Army of the North. But he was captured and imprisoned in Buda, Hungary. For three years Garnerin remained locked in a high tower, dreaming of escape. Like Bournonville, he thought a parachute was his only hope and passed his time designing parachutes. Garnerin had been making balloon ascensions since 1787, so he was not afraid of heights. Garnerin, though, was unable to get the materials he needed.

The Austrian campaign ended and Garnerin was released. He went back to Paris with his parachute designs. There he built a balloon and a parachute. On October 22, 1797, Garnerin was ready to make his first jump. His parachute, 23 feet in diameter, was shaped like a giant beach umbrella. It also folded up like one. A framework of 32 ribs was covered with canvas. Each rib was fastened at the top to a hoop that was attached to the net under the balloon.

At 6:00 P.M., André Garnerin climbed into the basket beneath the closed parachute. He slashed the ropes that held the balloon to the earth and began to climb. Up, up,

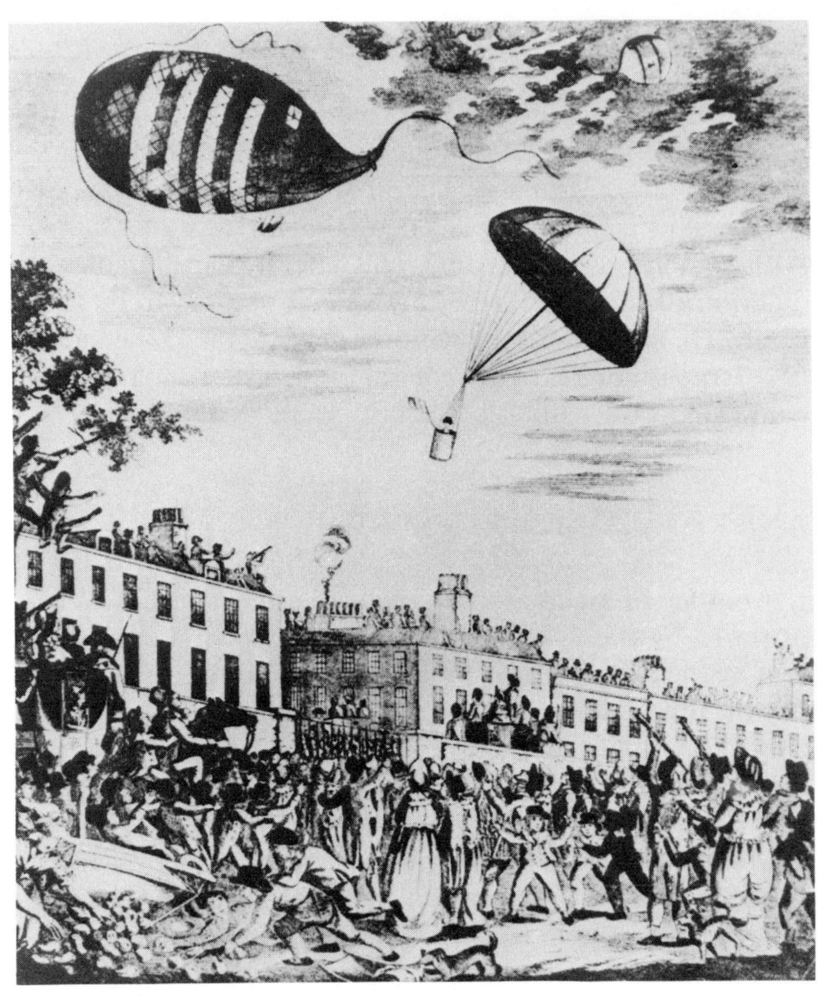

André Garnerin making the first parachute descent from a balloon, 1797

he went. There was a deep silence from the crowds of people gathered in the park to watch. This would be the first real parachute jump, and everyone thought Garnerin would be killed. At 3,000 feet he cut the cords that fastened the parachute to the balloon. Without his weight, the balloon shot up and exploded.

Garnerin's parachute, which had been closed, opened as

72

he descended. It came down much faster than expected. People screamed and ladies fainted, believing the brave parachutist was falling to his death. The parachute swung back and forth, or oscillated, wildly. Garnerin had to hold on to keep from being thrown out. This back-and-forth movement made Garnerin very seasick (perhaps we should say airsick). But he landed safely, mounted a horse, and rode back to the park. There he received a wild ovation from the waiting people.

Garnerin made several more parachute jumps in which the big umbrella oscillated in an alarming manner. The canopy had been coated so no air could pass through the fabric. Joseph Lalande, a French astronomer and friend of Garnerin, suggested he make a few holes to let some of the air spill out. Garnerin followed Lalande's suggestion, and the swaying motion was reduced. It was many years before parachutists found that a porous fabric, which let some air through, made for a more stable parachute.

In 1802, Garnerin went to London to make the first parachute jump in England. Spectators paid five shillings each to watch the spectacle at St. George's Parade. But it was impossible to keep the inhabitants of London, who had not paid, from watching. People clambered up every tree and structure to gain a vantage point. There were men sitting astride all the gabled roofs; others clung to chimneys.

By 5:15 P.M. on September 21, the huge striped balloon had been filled with hydrogen. The top of the parachute was then attached to the net covering the bag. The balloon was allowed to rise far enough to raise the parachute. The two towered 120 feet into the air. When all was ready, Garnerin climbed into the basket.

The cords were cut loose and the balloon began to rise. Garnerin was astonished when he saw the people packing the streets for miles around to see the event. They watched as Garnerin almost disappeared from view over Tottenham

Court Road. Then he cut the cords and the parachute began to descend.

The descent took about ten minutes. Thousands of people followed along on horseback under André. They held up their arms to him as if to catch him if he fell. For some reason Garnerin had chosen not to cut holes in this chute to allow air to spill out. He suffered for it. The basket swung so wildly it was, at times, higher than the chute.

André Garnerin made a safe landing and was instantly surrounded by thousands of enthusiastic people. Everyone wanted to embrace and congratulate him. The parachutist couldn't appreciate all this attention just then. He was violently airsick. The procession back to town had to make many stops because Garnerin was sick. He never made another parachute jump without air holes in his chute.

Garnerin's wife, Jeanne-Geneviève, joined him in making parachute descents. She had already made a name for herself as the first woman balloonist. Two years after André's first jump, she became the first woman to make a parachute descent. A few years later, Garnerin's niece, Eliza Garnerin, became the first professional woman parachutist. Between 1815 and 1836 she made forty jumps. She is credited with being the first person able to direct a parachute so as to land at a certain spot.

JORDAKI KUPARENTO

Jordaki Kuparento of Poland was the first aeronaut to make an emergency parachute jump. On July 24, 1808, Kuparento was giving a balloon exhibition over Warsaw. He rode beneath the parachute that was attached to the balloon. During one ascent, his hydrogen balloon burst into flames. The balloonist cut the parachute loose from the flaming mass and drifted safely to earth.

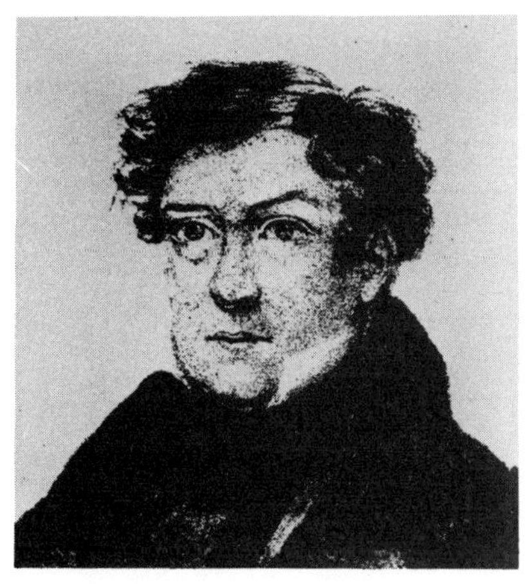

*Robert Cocking (1777–1837),
foolhardy parachutist*

ROBERT COCKING

When he was twenty-five, Robert Cocking watched André Garnerin's parachute descent in London. He was disturbed by the wild swinging of the parachute and felt it was due to the shape. The painter and balloon enthusiast resolved to design a parachute that would give a safe, comfortable ride.

Robert Cocking spent years studying parachutes. He tried and abandoned several designs. One day, while puzzling over the problem, he had a new idea. He took a parasol up to a second-floor balcony. Several times he dropped the parasol from the balcony, with the handle pointing downward. He found that the parasol always turned over in midair and landed handle up. From this experiment Cocking concluded that a parachute should be shaped like an inverted cone—or an upside-down parasol.

For many years Robert Cocking had to content himself with drawing designs and making model parachutes. He was not very successful as a painter and lacked the money to build a large parachute. After much thought, he went to see the proprietors of Vauxhall Gardens in London. These men owned the *Royal Nassau* balloon and used it in exhibitions. Cocking asked them to put up the money for him to build his parachute. In return, he promised, he would make a spectacular descent for them. The proprietors agreed to his suggestion. The jump turned out to be more spectacular than Cocking had planned.

Robert Cocking went to work and the parachute took shape. First he built a huge, saucer-shaped tin frame. This was covered with 124 square yards of Irish linen. A tin hoop, 34 feet in diameter, circled the parachute at its widest point. Painting decorated the underside. When finished, the parachute weighed 223 pounds. To this would be added Cocking's weight of 170 pounds. The *Royal Nassau,* the largest balloon in the world, was the only one large enough to lift this weight.

Some of Cocking's friends had doubts about the strength of the tin tubing. They felt ash wood would be stronger. Cocking would have none of this. He had full confidence in his parachute. Charles Green was to take the *Royal Nassau* up. He was very doubtful about this project. In the first place, he was worried about what would happen to the balloon when 400 pounds was dropped from it. In the second place, he wanted Cocking to test the parachute first with a dead weight. This Cocking refused to do.

The parachute descent was scheduled for July 24, 1837. It had taken thirty-five years for Cocking to see his dream come true. He was now, at age sixty-one, a little old for a parachute jump. But crowds of people came to Vauxhall Gardens to see it. This was the first parachute jump in England since André Garnerin's leap. The people expected to see another aerial triumph such as Garnerin had provided.

By five in the afternoon, the *Royal Nassau* bulged with gas. Charles Green and his assistant, Edward Spencer, got into the basket under the balloon. Then it was allowed to rise high enough so the open parachute could be attached.

76

Robert Cocking got into the wicker basket suspended under the parachute. Although short, stout, and elderly, the parachutist was dashing in a striped satin jacket and white trousers. He waved cheerfully to the huge crowds.

The ropes were cast off and the balloon and parachute rose majestically. The crowds cheered enthusiastically. Cocking had planned to descend from 8,000 feet. But in spite of numerous discharges of ballast, the balloon would only rise to 5,000 feet. It was carrying too much weight. Green called down to Cocking telling him he could go no higher.

"Well, I'll be leaving you then," said the plucky parachutist. "Good night, Mr. Green; good night, Mr. Spencer."

Robert Cocking cut the parachute loose. The balloon, freed of 400 pounds of weight, shot upward. According to Mr. Green they traveled "at the velocity of a sky-rocket."

No sooner had Cocking cut himself loose than the tin framework of the parachute began to crumple. The skeptics were right. The device was not strong enough. The canopy collapsed, and the brave but foolish inventor was carried to his death.

John Wise heard of Cocking's death. He studied the design of Cocking's parachute and believed it to be sound. On September 18, 1837, Wise ascended in his balloon to a half mile over Philadelphia. He carried with him two small test chutes, a dog, and a cat. First he tossed out a model of Garnerin's parachute attached to the yelping dog. It swung wildly all the way down. Next Wise tossed out the reluctant cat in a basket under a Cocking type of chute. It descended smoothly, although rotating slowly. The parachute landed on a rooftop and the cat took off for parts unknown. But Wise decided that the design of Cocking's parachute was sound but the tin framework had been too weak to support a man.

JOHN HAMPTON

The death of Robert Cocking caused a wave of public indignation. London newspapers were full of articles condemning such dangerous stunts. But, fifteen months later, John Hampton, a sailor and professional balloonist, was ready to make another jump. For safety he had modeled his parachute after the one used thirty-six years earlier by Garnerin. There was one difference. Garnerin's parachute opened after it was cut loose; Hampton's would already be open.

A few days before the jump, Hampton ran into trouble. There was a great deal of public feeling against the event. The owners of Montpellier Gardens, where the jump was to take place, realized they would be blamed if Hampton was killed. First, they decided to cancel the spectacle. But tickets had already been sold, and Hampton argued hard for the jump. At last the owners said they would allow him to make the descent on two conditions: that the balloon would be tethered and the jump would be made in the gardens.

Hampton agreed to these conditions in order to be allowed to make the descent. He probably never intended to stick to them.

The balloon ascent was to take place on October 3, 1838. In spite of the public outcry, the gardens were jammed. After the balloon was inflated and the parachute attached, a large coil of strong rope was tied to it. The twenty sturdy workmen holding on to the rope were told: "At all costs don't let go."

John Hampton got into the basket and waved cheerfully to the crowds. The men holding the rope slowly let the balloon rise to 40 feet. At this point, Hampton produced a knife and cut the rope. To the delight of the crowd, the balloon quickly climbed to 8,000 feet. Then Hampton used his knife again and cut the parachute free.

Without the weight of the parachute and man, the balloon rose rapidly. The bag burst right over Hampton's head with, as he said, "the violence of a thunderbolt." His parachute started floating downward gently without any dangerous oscillating. Hampton landed safely and became the first Englishman to make a successful parachute jump in England.

On June 13, 1839, John Hampton was to make a parachute descent in Cremorne Gardens. A huge crowd gathered for this event. By the time the balloon was inflated, it had become dangerously windy. Hampton announced that his jump would be postponed until the next day. The waiting people would have none of this. Hampton was forced to make the balloon ascent and parachute jump under very unfavorable conditions. He was blown against a wall and injured while landing.

John Hampton consistently overstated the danger of parachuting. According to him, the parachutist had difficulty breathing during a rapid drop. The only safe way to descend was with a large, rigid canopy to provide a slow descent. Such misconceptions were to persist for the next eighty years.

During the later half of the nineteenth century, parachutes were the toys of carnival aeronauts. In both Europe and America every circus and fair included a balloon ascension and a parachute descent. Crowds of people were attracted by these often dangerous performances. Stunts were performed to amuse the spectators. Acrobats hung by their knees from trapezes under parachutes. For eighty years little progress was made in chute design. All were rigid affairs, patterned after the one used by André Garnerin, and only suitable for use in calm weather. They were not seriously considered as an emergency device. There was no way a balloonist could stow one away and forget about it until it was needed.

THE FLEXIBLE PARACHUTE

Then, in 1880, a milestone in the history of parachuting was reached. For the first time a flexible parachute without a framework was used. The pressure of the air filled it out as it descended. This new, flexible parachute was still tied under a balloon to be cut loose when needed.

Who invented the flexible parachute? Well, it was one of two men. One was an American, Captain Tom Baldwin. The other was Captain P. A. Van Tassell, a Dutchman who had settled in the United States. Although Baldwin has generally received credit for the chute, Van Tassell was probably the originator. He tutored Baldwin and taught him all he knew about parachuting. Later both men began to use the flexible chute and both claimed to have invented it.

The first flexible chute used by Van Tassell was not very impressive. The canopy was merely a round piece of cotton cloth. Later, stronger and lighter silk was used. Cords were fastened around the perimeter of the chute and a trapeze was hung from them. Friends of Van Tassell were appalled to hear that he planned to risk his life by hanging from this piece of cloth.

Captain Van Tassell made his first jump over a cow pasture outside of Los Angeles in the early 1880s. The Dutchman did not lack courage. He weighed over two hundred pounds and the flexible parachute had never been tested.

After the balloon ascended to 4,000 feet, Van Tassell climbed onto the trapeze, which hung 15 feet below the parachute. Then he cut himself loose from the balloon. His friends on the ground watched fearfully, expecting him to come plummeting down. But the slack canopy swelled out at once as the parachute began to drop. Van Tassell landed safely after a smooth ride.

Captain Baldwin's parachute was almost identical to the

one made by Van Tassell. Later, he developed a body harness to which the parachute was attached. Baldwin was more of a showman and so became better known. He gave exhibitions of parachute jumping all over the world. The Prince of Wales, later King Edward VII, asked Baldwin to give a command parachuting performance for the royal family.

When the nineteenth century closed, the sole use of parachutes was for entertainment. But early in the twentieth century an event occurred that was soon to cause all high flyers to take another look at the parachute.

6. 1900 TO 1918

THE INVENTION OF THE AIRPLANE

Thursday, December 17, 1903, was windy and cold. The puddles from the rain a few days before were now coated with ice. The vacationists had all gone home. There was little to do at Kitty Hawk, North Carolina, at this time of year. The men not on duty at the Kill Devil Hill Life Saving Station were sitting around, idle. Then one of them picked up the binoculars and trained them on the dunes about a mile away.

"Hurrah!" he shouted. "There's a flag flying over at the Wright brothers' camp. They're going to try for a flight today."

At this announcement the six off-duty men reached for their jackets. Everyone at the Life Saving Station had become a fan of the two brothers who were experimenting on the sand dunes of Kitty Hawk. The men helped Wilbur and Orville move their 605-pound aircraft when necessary. The brothers appreciated their help and, in return, always put up a flag when they were going to try to make a flight.

On December 17, Wilbur and Orville Wright had been at their camp at Kitty Hawk for eighty-four days. They were all out of food except for beans. The weather was growing steadily worse, and they were expected home for

Christmas in Dayton, Ohio, in a week. This would have to be their last try of the year.

In their experiments, the brothers took turns acting as pilot. Monday had been Wilbur's turn. That attempt never got off the ground. Orville would have the first turn today. The brothers had built a track to use in launching their craft on the soft sand. Orville got on the machine at 10:34 A.M. and began warming up the engine and propeller. The rope was cast off and the craft started down the track. Wilbur ran alongside, holding on to the right wing. The machine lifted from the track before it reached the end. John T. Daniel, from the Life Saving Station, snapped a picture of this historic flight with a camera set up by the Wrights. This flight lasted only 12 seconds and covered 120 feet. Several more trials were made that day. On the fourth and last trip, the plane covered 852 feet in 59 seconds. The age of powered flight had arrived.

Although the first beginnings were feeble, progress was rapid. Two years later the Wright brothers could keep an airplane in the air for as long as thirty-nine minutes. In Europe and America, other inventors were experimenting with new airplane designs.

Did parachutists see a new opportunity in this revolutionary mode of aerial transportation? They did not. A decade after the first powered flight, parachutists thought anyone who would jump from an airplane must be crazy. In the first place, airplanes didn't fly high enough for a parachute to be be needed. In the second place, parachutes were fine for a jump from a slow-moving balloon—but a jump from an airplane traveling at thirty or forty miles per hour? It wasn't to be thought of. The canopy would be torn to shreds. The shroud lines would become entangled with the airplane. Then the airman would be dragged to a certain death. These thoughts prevented parachutes from being considered for jumps from airplanes.

TWO BRAVE WOMEN

So, at the start of the twentieth century, parachutists were jumping from balloons. Thus far we haven't mentioned the many women among these early twentieth-century parachutists. Let's tell the harrowing story of two of these brave women.

Daisy Sheppard and Louise May were going to perform a twin parachute jump over Staffordshire, England, in 1908. This was Louise May's first jump. At first everything went well. The balloon ascended with the two women riding under the two parachutes on trapezes about five feet apart. At 4,000 feet, Daisy said to Louise, "As this is your first jump, I want you to pull your rope and start down first."

Louise pulled and tugged, but the rope was tangled and she couldn't release her parachute. Following Daisy's instructions, Louise tried to climb up to release it. She lacked the strength.

All this time the balloon was rising rapidly. They were now at well over 7,000 feet. Daisy could have cut herself loose and saved her own life. But if she did that, Louise would be carried so high she would die from lack of oxygen or would be blown out to sea. Daisy chose to stay with Louise and try to save her.

Next Daisy and Louise tried to swing their trapezes so Louise could reach the one Daisy was on. This didn't work. Then the balloon entered a cloud. They were now over two miles above the earth and still rising.

Probably not being able to see the earth far below gave Louise the courage to do a very brave thing. She jumped the five feet to Daisy's trapeze. Louise landed on Daisy's knees, but slipped down until she only held on to Daisy's ankle by one hand. With Daisy's help she managed to crawl up until they were both on the trapeze under Daisy's parachute.

Daisy pulled the rope and the parachute dropped. But it

was not completely open and fell very rapidly. The women landed, with Louise on top of Daisy. Louise May escaped injury in her terrifying first parachute jump. Daisy wasn't so lucky. The rough landing resulted in paralysis of her spine. But within a few weeks she was making plans for more parachute jumps.

So, at the start of the twentieth century, the time still wasn't ripe for parachute jumps from airplanes. In addition, these early airplane pilots were not overly concerned with safety. They just wanted to get their machines into the air and keep them there. In the first ten years of powered flight, more than three hundred pilots were killed in crashes. This is a lot when you consider how few airplanes there were then. After a while, one fact could not be ignored. A safe parachute jump can be made from 300 feet. Two out of five of the pilots fell 300 feet or more to their death. If a way could be found to use parachutes in airplanes, many lives could be saved.

RALPH CARHART

Designers of parachutes, although not intending them for use with airplanes, were not idle. There were a few innovations. In 1905, Ralph Carhart jumped from a balloon using his own free type of parachute. It was carried in a pack worn on the chest. The canopy was folded up and a small pilot chute was laid on top of it. The entire pack was held shut by safety pins. After Carhart jumped, he unfastened the safety pins. Then the pilot chute tugged the larger one out of the pack. The entire affair was rather primitive, but it seems to have worked.

CHARLES BROADWICK

Charles Broadwick was always dreaming up ways to thrill the public. He devised a way to hide his parachute from his audience when jumping from a balloon. It was folded up and placed in a bag sewn into the back of a vest he wore. A thin cord, invisible from the ground, was fastened from the basket to the top of the canopy. When Broadwick jumped, onlookers could not see the parachute. People screamed, expecting him to fall to his death. After Broadwick had fallen a short distance, the static line pulled the canopy out of the pack and he floated down safely. Broadwick used this vest-pack parachute in hundreds of jumps.

FIRST JUMP FROM AN AIRPLANE

At this time it was believed that the loss of weight when a parachutist jumped would throw an airplane out of control. Pilots, as well as parachutists, were very reluctant to try this stunt. But someone finally did get up the courage to make the first big jump.

Captain Albert Berry is generally credited with being the first person to make a parachute jump from an airplane. Berry was the son of a balloonist and was himself a professional jumper. He was not, as has sometimes been reported, a captain in the U. S. Army. For some unknown reason all parachutists then were called "captain." As the first jump was made at an Army base, some people supposed Berry to be an Army captain.

Anyway, in early 1912, Thomas Benoist, who operated an aviation school in St. Louis, Missouri, wanted some publicity. He decided that the first parachute jump from an airplane should do the trick. Albert Berry agreed to make the jump.

A galvanized-iron cone was fastened to the undercarriage of the biplane to carry the parachute. Both Berry and the pilot, Anthony Jannus, would ride in open seats. When it was time for Berry to jump, he would climb down onto the axle, fasten on the parachute, and jump.

Twice the two men went up to make the jump. Both times poor weather forced them to cancel it. On March 1, 1912, they went up for the third time. The jump was scheduled to be held at Jefferson Barracks, seventeen miles from St. Louis. It took the airplane a half hour to cover this distance with the two men riding in the open. The weather was freezing and a light snow drifted down. Berry was stiff with cold when he climbed down onto the axle and fastened on the chute.

The soldiers below watched as the little biplane circled the barracks at an altitude of 1,500 feet and a speed of 55 miles per hour. Then they saw a man drop from the plane. To the surprise of everyone, the airplane continued to fly straight and level.

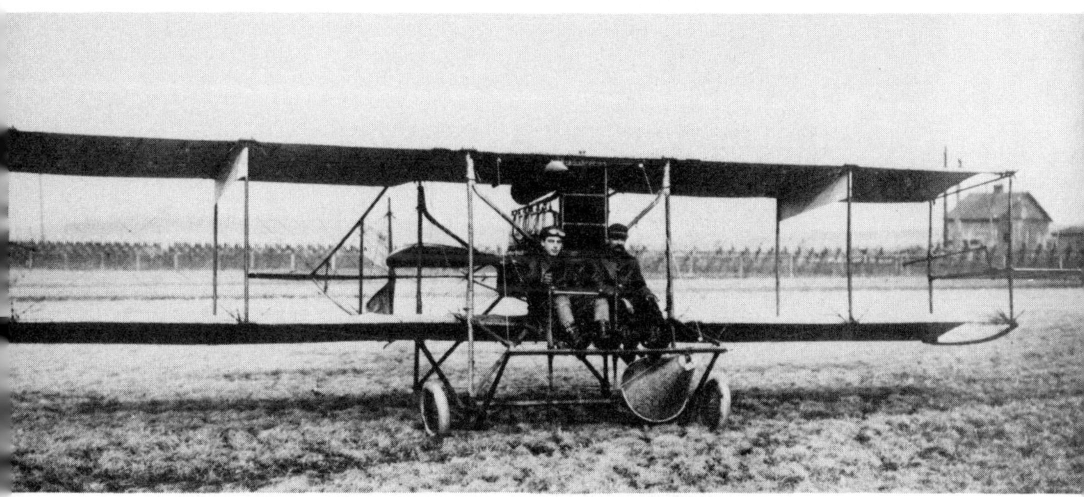

Albert Berry and pilot before first parachute jump in 1912

Berry dropped about five hundred feet before the canopy of his chute opened. There was a bad moment when the stiff wind almost slammed him into the mess hall. Captain Berry pulled up his feet and just grazed the top of the building. He landed safely in a field beyond.

No one thought this first jump from an airplane of much importance. The commander of the Army base didn't bother to watch it. Benoist didn't get there until it was all over. To Berry, it was just another stunt, like the jumps he usually made from balloons.

Albert Berry repeated the jump on March 10, 1912. The weather then was worse. It was bitterly cold and snowing hard. The cloud deck was at less than 1,000 feet. The airplane had to fly under these clouds. Berry jumped from an altitude of 800 feet.

The wind was so stiff it blew the jumper and chute up and down. At times Berry was higher than his canopy. The wind nearly blew him into a clump of trees. But Berry tugged at the shroud lines and managed to land in a snowy field. His face was blue from cold. When asked if he planned on making another jump, he replied, "Not unless they pay me a lot more money."

FIRST JUMP FROM A HYDROPLANE

Frederick Rodman Law was a steeplejack. He made his living painting and repairing flagpoles and steeples. When he could find work, he spent his days at dizzying heights.

But business was bad. Few had heard of Frederick Law, steeplejack. He tried to think of some way to attract attention. A parachute jump seemed like the answer.

On February 2, 1912, a group of school children visited the Statue of Liberty. They stood in front of the statue as the teacher began to read Emma Lazarus' poem.

"Look, look," yelled a boy. "There is a man up there."

"He's going to jump," screamed a little girl.

The teacher and children looked up to see a man climbing over the railing around the torch. As they watched, he jumped. Halfway down, a big striped canopy opened. The breeze caught the chute and blew it toward a granite coping. The man landed against it with a thump.

When the children rushed over, Frederick Law was gathering up his parachute. Then he limped off to collect $1,500 from a newsreel company that filmed the jump from a boat. Law decided that parachuting paid better than steeplejacking.

A short time later Fred Law jumped off the East River Bridge with a parachute. He landed among the ice floes in the river and was fished out, blue with cold. A film crew paid him for doing that stunt. A little later Law jumped off the Bankers Trust Building on Wall Street. By now the newspapers were calling him Fearless Frederick.

Next, Law was asked to make a jump from a hydroplane over Marblehead, Massachusets. On April 13, 1912, he was to use and demonstrate a parachute developed by H. Leo Stevens. It was one of the first knapsack type of chutes. The canopy was packed into a container that was attached to a leather harness. The jumper wore the harness throughout the jump. A static line tied from the wing strut to the canopy would pull the chute from the container when the parachutist jumped. Fifty thousand people watched as the pilot climbed to 1,500 feet. Everything went smoothly on the first hydroplane jump.

Things did not go smoothly for Fearless on his next stunt. He was hired to be the first astronaut. The first spaceship for manned flight, a huge skyrocket, had been built. A "control room" was provided for Fearless to protect him from "G-forces." It sat atop 50 pounds of slow-burning black powder that was to boost Fearless 3,500 feet skyward. He was to return by parachute.

The rocket was mounted on top of a 25-foot gantry. Law

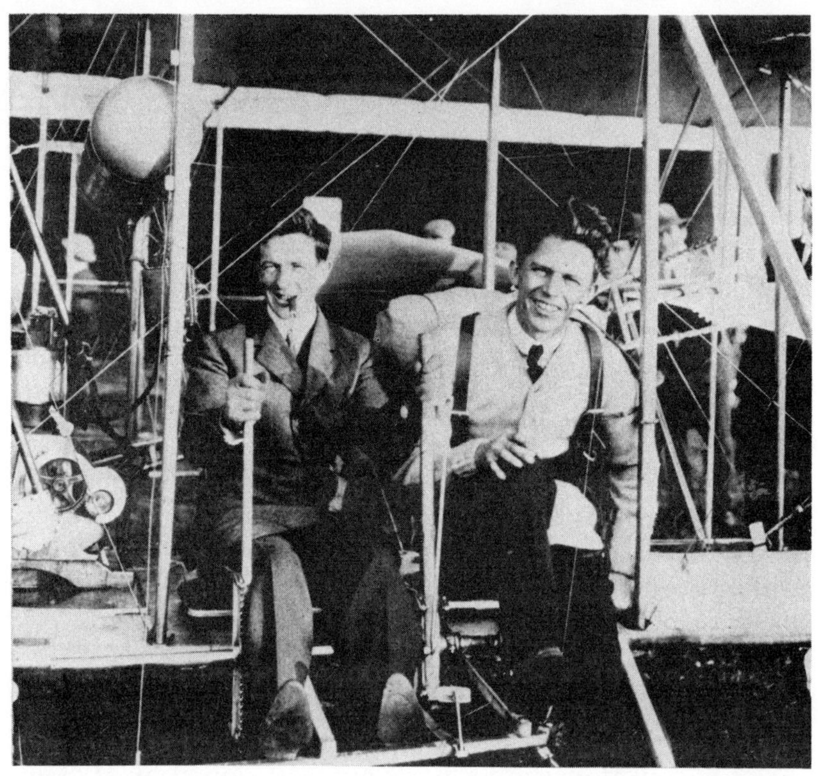

Frederick Rodman Law before his first parachute jump

waved to the crowds, put on his football helmet, and climbed the ladder to his "control room." After the hatch was closed, an attendant lit the fuse. Then he ran for his life. As the fuse hissed, the newsreel cameras began to turn, ready to record the first space flight.

Then a terrific explosion knocked the spectators to the ground. The camera crew was flattened. Splintered wood and shreds of metal flew in all directions. A great orange ball of fire engulfed poor Law. His body shot up into the air and then came down with a thud.

People ran to the would-be astronaut, expecting to find him dead. But after a few moments, Fearless came to. He sat up, grinned, and asked, "What happened?"

FIRST WOMAN TO JUMP FROM AN AIRPLANE

Georgia Thompson "Tiny" Broadwick made her first parachute jump from a hot-air balloon when she was fifteen. For years after this she toured the fair circuit with her foster father, Charles Broadwick. He was a pioneer in parachuting and developed one of the first backpack chutes.

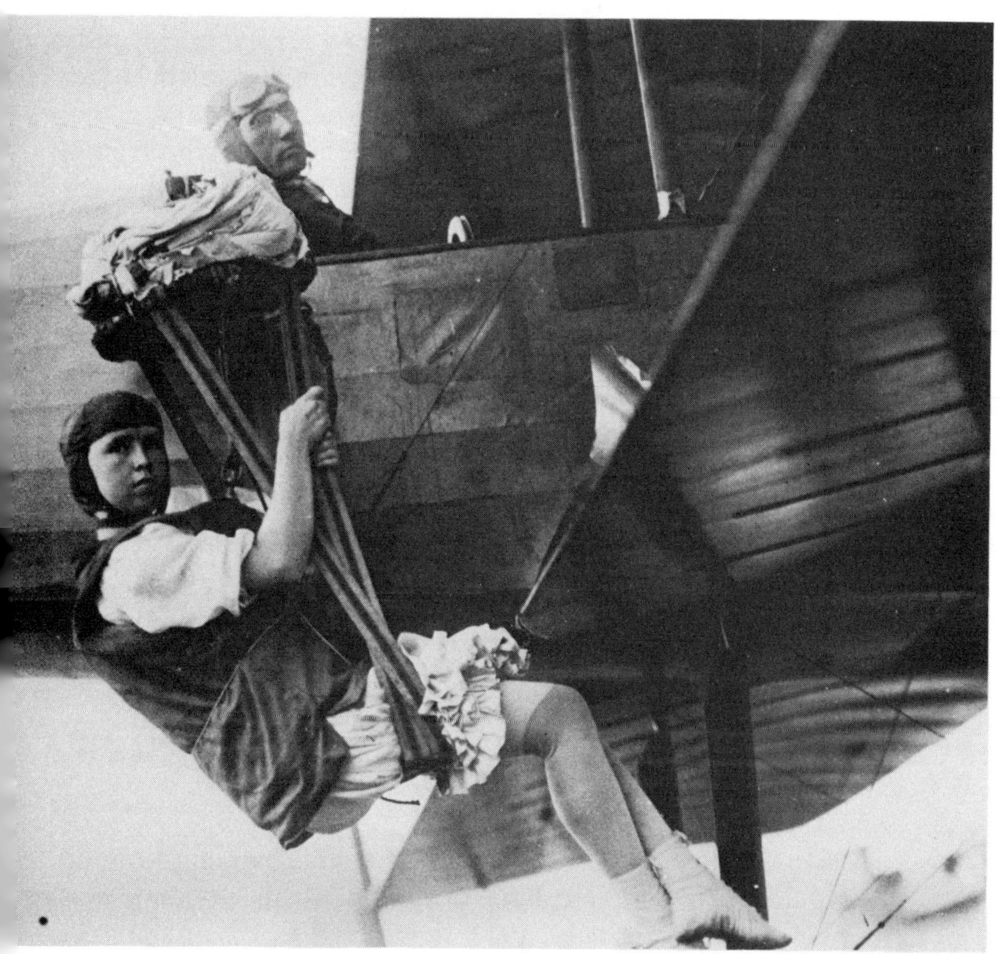

Tiny Broadwick about to jump
from Martin airplane, 1913

Although only fifteen at the time of her first jump, Tiny was already a self-assured young woman. She was married and had a baby. For her parachuting exhibitions, she used the name Tiny Broadwick.

When Tiny made her first jumps, she was billed as "The Doll." It is easy to see why. She was 5 feet tall and weighed 80 pounds. During exhibitions she wore shoulder-length curls and frilly dresses and tights.

On June 21, 1913, at Los Angeles, Tiny Broadwick became the first woman to jump from an airplane. Her pilot for this and many other jumps was Glen L. Martin. Later he was to become a leader in the aircraft industry.

Also in 1913, Tiny was the first woman to jump from a hydroplane. In 1914, she was the first person of either sex to give an official demonstration of parachutes for the Federal Government. As a result, several of Broadwick's safety-pack chutes were ordered by the U.S. Army for further testing. During Tiny's jumping career of fourteen years, she made 1,100 jumps safely.

After 1914, Tiny always wore her foster father's "Patent Safety-Pack Vest" for her jumps. At one time it saved her life. In 1915, Tiny was taking part in an aerial display at the World's Fair in San Francisco. The wings on the airplane in which she was riding came off in midair. Tiny jumped and landed safely. The pilot wore no chute and was killed in the crash.

FIRST PARACHUTE JUMP FROM AN AIRPLANE IN EUROPE

In Europe it was still believed that a parachute jump would throw an airplane out of control. A jump was planned for August 19, 1913, in which the pilot and jumper would be the same person. The parachute would be opened by a spring-loading device while the airplane was under way. The canopy would billow out and pull the pilot out of the cockpit. Then the airplane would be allowed to crash. Everything worked as planned for the pilot, Adolphe Pégoud. He made a safe, if rather uncomfortable, landing in the top of a tree.

The action of the airplane after he left it fascinated Pégoud and all observers. Without a pilot, the airplane continued to fly smoothly. It performed a loop-the-loop and landed safely.

This was the first time anyone had seen an airplane do this trick. Adolphe Pégoud took the airplane back up and tried a loop-the-loop. It worked so well it became one of his usual stunts. He was the first man to perform an aerial loop-the-loop.

WORLD WAR I

As World War I approached, the parachute, it would seem, would be a lifesaver. This was not so. The refusal to recognize the potential of the parachute, at least in hindsight, seems unbelievable. Less than a year before the outbreak of the war, England's Royal Flying Corps declared: "Frankly, we see very little future for the parachute as a lifesaving apparatus in emergency on aeroplanes." The military felt that the purpose of wartime aircraft was to fight, not to serve as platforms for parachute jumpers. There was a general feeling that a parachute might cause a pilot to abandon his aircraft without sufficient cause. Airmen themselves felt that only a coward would wear a parachute.

It must be admitted that there were still problems in jumping from an airplane with a parachute. Rip cords were not in general use then. The jumper could not delay the opening of the parachute until clear of the airplane. There was always danger of the chute or shroud lines becoming entangled with the falling aircraft.

Observation Balloons

"Look over there toward Rheims, Sydney," said James Webb. "I think the Huns are on the march."

Sydney trained his telescope on the road. Now he caught the glint of metal from the rifles carried by the marching troops. "You're right, James. That is what the Major wanted to know." He picked up the field telephone.

James Webb and Sydney Paine spent their days in an observation balloon tethered high over the Allied lines. In the distance the French countryside lay in a checkered green pattern. But below them everything was devastated. The earth was pockmarked with bomb craters. The few trees still standing were twisted and splintered. A line of bare dirt marked the front line held by the British. This was World War I. The Germans and the Allies were locked in deadly trench warfare. Thousands of lives were expended to gain or lose a few yards.

James kept his binoculars trained on the distant troops. Headquarters would want to know their number and destination. He did not hear the distant buzz that grew ever louder.

"It's a German Fokker headed this way," yelled Sydney.

James wheeled around. He wasn't too surprised. They both knew the Germans would try to keep the movements of their troops from being observed. The Fokker was headed directly toward them. There was no time to lose. The two men wore their harnesses with the shroud lines attached. Their parachutes, packed in conical bags, hung over the sides of the basket. As the Fokker opened fire, Sydney went over one side while James went over the other.

Before the men hit the ground, the incendiary bullets from the machine guns had ignited the hydrogen in the balloon. The flaming mass collapsed onto the basket. But Sydney and James would be back up the next day, observ-

94

ing from a different balloon.

Observation balloons were widely used in World War I. A vast strip of devastation, no-man's-land, stretched between the entrenched enemies. Balloons served as platforms from which observers could watch the enemy's movements. But each side was very successful in shooting down the other's balloons. The tethered bags were an easy target for low-flying aircraft. At the start of the war, the death rate among balloon observers was enormous. They were the first to be issued parachutes for use while aloft.

Parachutes were soon being used in other ways in World War I. Small parachutes carrying magnesium flares were dropped at night to illuminate target areas. Spies regularly parachuted in behind the enemy lines. Black canopies were used at night to decrease the risk of their being spotted.

Aircraft

By this time parachutes were fairly reliable. But the first combat airmen had more bravado than brains. They didn't use them. When hit by enemy fire, the pilot had two choices. He could either jump and be killed or try to ride the plane down and be cremated. Over six thousand British pilots died because of lack of parachutes.

One case of this type was Major Raoul Lufbery, the American commander of the 94th Aero Squadron. He led Eddie Rickenbacker and others over enemy lines to give them their first taste of air battle.

Major Lufbery trained many pilots. Before going into combat, they always asked the question that was on all of their minds. "What do you do, Major, if your plane catches fire?"

The major always answered, "You sideslip. The wind may put the fire out, and it keeps the flames from blowing back at you. Just remember, whatever you do, don't panic and jump. Ride your ship down and you'll have a chance of flying again."

On May 19, 1918, Lufbery led a patrol of new flyers. During combat the major's aircraft was hit and burst into flames. Lufbery was seen peering over the side as he used his arms to try to protect his face from the searing flames. Then the major ignored his own advice. He couldn't stand the heat. He crawled out on the wing and jumped to coolness and death.

The terrible toll in airmen resulted in an increase in parachute experiments—especially in Britain. The "Guardian Angel" chute developed by Everard Calthrop showed the most promise. But, as it was stored outside the airplane, it was vulnerable to enemy fire. The view of the British Air Ministry still was "Parachutes are impractical."

In 1918, the Air Ministry got a nasty jolt. For some time there had been rumors that German pilots were using parachutes. This was not believed. But now three cases of escapes by German pilots wearing parachutes were confirmed. In addition, an American pursuit force shot down eleven German airplanes. All eleven pilots landed safely with parachutes. Soon after this a German parachute was recovered. It consisted of a canopy stuffed into a sack. The pilot sat upon it during flight, wearing a harness to which shroud lines were attached. A static line was used to deploy the chute when he jumped.

The fact that German aviators were wearing parachutes impressed the Allies. In England the process of finding a safe parachute was speeded up. In the closing days of World War I, a few Allied airmen were saved by using parachutes. But the adoption of parachutes came too late to save thousands of pilots.

7. FREE FALL FOR ALL

McCOOK FLYING FIELD

The biplane circled and came back over the airfield at an altitude of 1,500 feet. The figure of a man came hurtling out of the plane, followed by the shroud lines of a parachute. The canopy, packed under the fuselage, broke loose and opened. The five men on the ground watched intently. Now and then one of them made a note on the pad of paper in his hand.

The jumper landed with a thump on the edge of the runway. The men paid no attention to the still figure. All eyes were on the airplane as it circled the field again. Now a new parachute and jumper came floating down. Soon another quiet figure was lying in a field to the left of the runway. The men paid no attention to that one, either, as they made notes.

"Well, let's go inside and talk this over," said the Major. He seemed to be the senior officer in charge of the group. "Sergeant Fulton, have someone pick up those chutes and dummies. We'll use them again tomorrow."

Soon the five men were gathered around a table in the barracks, discussing the results of the tests with the Mears parachute from Britain. These tests took place at McCook Flying Field in Dayton, Ohio, in 1919. A research center for parachute development had been set up there near the end of World War I. From this center came the modern parachute.

What happened to the parachute when World War I finally came to a close? Except in the United States, very little. Without a war to spur them on, most countries lost interest in parachute research. Fortunately, this was not the case in the United States. The U.S. Army was anxious to develop an air corps. Already a huge investment in trained pilots had been made. Now some insurance for these pilots was needed. The Army wanted to be sure that, in most cases, these airmen could walk away from an airplane crash. Funds were earmarked for parachute development.

On January 1, 1919, a research center was set up at McCook Flying Field. Major E. L. Hoffman, an aeronautical engineer, was put in charge. From all over the United States, he gathered together a group of men dedicated to parachuting.

The question sometimes arises as to who first invented and tried out many of the parachuting improvements now in use. This is often difficult to tell. The early parachutists made and designed their own parachutes. They borrowed ideas from each other. Often an inventor didn't bother to patent an idea. This didn't seem important then. Sometimes an idea was adopted and patented by another jumper. But all these brave jumpers contributed to the development of the parachute.

At McCook, the scientific approach was applied to solving the problem of a safe parachute. Samples of chutes were obtained from all over the world. Almost all parachutes in use then were attached to the airplane. The jumper wore a harness to which the shroud lines were fastened. These parachutes were tested, using dummies, in all types of conditions. All jumps were studied and discussed. After the tests were completed, the group at McCook decided that attached parachutes were not suitable for jumps from airplanes. They set up a list of strict requirements for the ideal parachute. Only those parachutes that met the requirements were considered.

Under the leadership of Major Hoffman, the group went to work to design the ideal parachute. Ideas were proposed by all participants and tested. As a result of this effort, the "A" type of free-fall parachute was developed. This chute was packed into a bag that was attached to the back of the harness worn by the jumper. After the pilot jumped, he pulled a hand-operated rip cord that opened the flap on the pack. A small auxiliary parachute was on top of the large chute. It opened and pulled the large chute out of the pack.

Floyd Smith was one of the group working at McCook. He was already a pilot and a designer of parachutes. Smith was responsible for the design of the first practical free-fall parachute.

By April 1919, Major Hoffman believed they were ready to test their ideal parachute in a "live" jump. Leslie Leroy Irvin, one of the McCook group, was asked to make the first jump. Irvin was a former circus performer and parachutist. At this time, it was generally believed that a free fall would cause the jumper to lose consciousness. For that reason not many parachutists wanted to make such a jump. But one of Irvin's circus stunts had been a leap without a parachute from a high platform into a net far below. Irvin had performed this trick many times. It convinced him that a free fall would not make a jumper lose consciousness.

On April 19, 1919, Irvin went up for the test, with Floyd Smith as his pilot. Irvin jumped and let himself drop 1,000 feet. Then he pulled the rip cord, the canopy opened, and he sailed smoothly down. This first free-fall jump so excited Irvin that he was careless in landing and broke an ankle. But Irvin wasn't killed, and he didn't lose consciousness. The Army gave Irvin a contract to build three hundred of these parachutes.

The McCook group went on experimenting in an effort

to solve other parachuting problems. In spite of the work at McCook, the majority of airmen all over the world still believed in the superiority of the attached chute. The McCook group wondered what arguments they could use to convince them. As it turned out, they didn't have to use any arguments. Several disasters, or near-disasters, occurred in rapid succession. The first two involved attached parachutes. These accidents helped convince airmen of the superiority of the Irvin chute.

The first accident was a picture-taking flight, over Chicago, of the hydrogen blimp, the *Wing Foot Express*. All five men on board were provided with parachutes carried in bags attached to the outside of the basket. At five in the afternoon the *Wing Foot Express* suddenly burst into flames. All five of the attached parachute canopies were burned—some more than others. Only two men made it safely to the ground. The canopies of the other three were too burned to support the men.

A short time later the British government sent Lieutenant R. A. Caldwell to McCook Field to demonstrate their Guardian Angel parachute. This chute was then used by many pilots in the Royal Air Force. The British hoped to convince the U.S. Army of the superiority of their own attached type of parachute. They also hoped to find a market for their chute in the United States. For this jump, the canopy, as usual, was fastened under the fuselage. The lines from the canopy went up to the harness worn by Caldwell in the cockpit. When the lieutenant jumped, the shroud lines became hooked on an elevator rocker arm. Caldwell dangled helplessly below the airplane. Within a few seconds, the sharp rocker arm had sawed the shroud lines in two. Without a canopy, Caldwell plunged to his death before the horrified Army officials he had hoped to convince. The death of Caldwell killed belief in the superiority of the attached parachute.

The Irvin chute also received a boost from a near-accident. LeRoy B. Jahn had developed a quick-opening parachute. The canopy on his chute contained built-in springs, which, according to the inventor, snapped the canopy open quickly after the parachutist jumped. He came to McCook Field hoping to convince the Army that his parachute was superior to theirs. He brought William O'Conner along to make the jump. Everyone at McCook was still shocked by the death of Caldwell and didn't want the tragedy repeated. Major Hoffman decided they would watch this demonstration on one condition. O'Conner would have to wear an Irvin parachute as a safety precaution in addition to the Jahn chute. This condition made Jahn very angry. He accused them of insulting his parachute. But the Army was firm. There would be no demonstration unless O'Conner also wore one of their chutes.

O'Conner finally went up wearing two parachutes. At 2,000 feet he jumped. Then, as the horrified spectators watched, he plummeted down for 1,500 feet, with the Jahn parachute flapping uselessly overhead. At 500 feet, O'Conner finally pulled the rip cord on the Irvin chute. It opened quickly and brought him down safely. This test served to convince the Army of only one thing. They already had the best parachute. In the first three years of use, it saved forty-two lives.

Hoffman and his group next came up with the simplified "type S" parachute. This was the forerunner of all modern emergency and sport parachutes.

By this time, parachutes, although not required, were available for use to members of the Air Corps. Most pilots chose not to be bothered. But safety was soon to be tightened. At Air Corps bases, on January 15, 1922, pilots gathered around bulletin boards. They stared in disbelief at an order issued by General Billy Mitchell, Chief of the Air Corps:

"Henceforth, service type parachutes will be worn
by all military flying personnel."

A short time later the British Royal Air Force adopted the McCook type of parachute for use by their pilots. The attached parachute was forgotten.

THE CATERPILLAR CLUB

Do you want to belong to the most exclusive club in the world? You don't have to be wealthy or well known to join. Members come from every walk of life. There is only one requirement. You must have saved your own life by having jumped with a parachute.

The first member was Lieutenant Harold R. Harris. On October 20, 1922, Harris took off from McCook Field to test an experimental fighting plane. At 2,500 feet the wings came off. Lieutenant Harris had never made a parachute jump and didn't much want to make this one. When the young officer stood up in the cockpit, the rushing slipstream snatched him out. Harris began a long, uncontrolled free fall. Three times he jerked on a strap, but nothing happened. At 500 feet the despairing pilot finally realized he was pulling on his leg strap. He pulled the rip cord, and the chute opened and brought him down safely.

Two newspapermen, Maurice Hutton and Verne Timmerman, interviewed Harris about his jump. They decided there should be a club for airmen who had saved their lives by jumping. They coined the name Caterpillar Club because parachute canopies then were made of silk woven by caterpillars. Ironically, both men missed their one chance of becoming members of the club they helped to form. Three years later Hutton and Timmerman were killed in an airplane crash. Neither was wearing a parachute.

In 1924, another airman joined the Caterpillars. Lieutenant Frank Tyndall had the wings ripped off his Martin 3-A bomber in a storm near Seattle, Washington. He too saved himself by jumping.

Charles A. Lindbergh saved himself with a parachute on four different occasions. It takes a lot of luck to survive four airplane crashes. These jumps earned him the nickname of Lucky Lindy.

The Caterpillar Club now has more than thirty thousand members. It is estimated, though, that as many as one hundred thousand people are eligible to belong. Leslie Irvin kept the records of the Caterpillars until his death in 1966. He sent a gold pin to each new member. After his death, his widow continued the work.

HIGH JUMPERS

At the start of the 1920s, aircraft were of the low-performance type. All flew low and slow. Then, as pilots gained confidence and airplanes were improved, they began to fly at higher altitudes. Now a new question came up. Could a parachute be used at these higher altitudes? At that time there was a general belief that parachutes would not function in the rarefied atmosphere at 20,000 feet. Sergeant Ralph Bottriel of the Army research team at McCook Field did not believe this. His reasoning was that as the air at four or five miles could support an airplane, it should also open a parachute and uphold a man.

On June 28, 1921, Bottriel went up to make the test. An unfortunate accident nearly ended his life. Before making the jump, Bottriel stood up in the rear cockpit of the biplane at 20,500 feet. While trying to signal the pilot, he accidentally pulled the rip cord.

The canopy opened with such force that Bottriel was jerked from the cockpit. His body crashed through the tail section, shattering and cutting his left arm. The sergeant was weak from shock, lack of oxygen and blood. His left arm was bleeding profusely. He managed to wrap a shroud line around his left arm for a tourniquet while descending.

Bottriel's record for a scientific, high-altitude jump stood for three years. Then Captain A. W. Stevens of McCook Field jumped safely from 26,500 feet.

Another big question at this time was whether or not a jumper would become unconscious during a long free fall. Sergeant Randall Bose, in 1924, made several drops of 1,500 to 2,000 feet. During one of these, he discovered the lethal trap in free falls. On this jump he went into what is now known as a deadly flat spin. Centrifugal force during one of these spins causes the blood to pool in the head and extremities. This results in a curtain of redness before the eyes. The heart and lungs do not get sufficient blood. If the spin continues, the jumper loses consciousness. Fortunately Sergeant Bose pulled his rip cord before he blacked out.

In 1925, an Army instructor, Steven Budreau, demonstrated that spin could be eliminated if the jumper "stabilized" himself through body position. A spread-eagle position, with arms and legs extended back, would keep the jumper from spinning. He fell from 7,000 feet to 3,500 feet while under perfect control.

In 1941, World War II had already begun. The U. S. Air Corps needed to know if it was safe for a jumper to make even longer free falls. During combat, a pilot descending by parachute was a sitting duck for enemy fire. If he could delay the opening of his parachute until he was close to the ground, he would have a better chance to survive. The Air Corps asked Arthur H. Starnes to make a jump for them.

Arthur Starnes had begun making delayed drops in 1925. He developed his jumping technique until he could jump from 10,000 feet and only open his chute a few hundred feet above the ground. His jump in 1941, for the Air Corps, was his greatest performance and the first notable scientific free fall. The jumper carried 100 pounds of instruments to record scientific information. Starnes fell from 30,800 feet to 1,500 feet. The shock caused by the opening parachute was greater than had been expected. Starnes blacked out. But the Air Corps found out what they wanted to know. A pilot could free fall thousands of feet and survive.

Three of the most incredible parachute jumps of all time were performed by Captain Joseph W. Kittenger, Jr. These were made as part of Project Excelsior. This was a high-altitude survival program aimed at developing equipment and techniques for airmen forced to abandon their aerospace crafts. Kittenger's jumps were made from an open balloon gondola. Jumps of 76,400 feet, 75,000 feet, and 102,800 feet were made. On his last jump, from nearly twenty miles up, the free fall lasted for 4½ minutes. Kittenger dropped 84,800 feet before opening his chute at 18,000 feet. During this fall, his body traveled at a speed of 614 miles per hour.

WORLD WAR II

By 1944, the tide of war was turning. Early in the war, London received nightly poundings from Hitler's *Luftwaffe*. Now the British Royal Air Force was sending waves of bombers across the channel every night to bomb Berlin's war industries.

Flight Sergeant Nicholas Alkemade was in good humor as he prepared for the nightly bombing run. This would be his thirteenth and last run over Berlin. Sunday he was going on leave. At dusk he greeted the other six members of the crew of the Lancaster bomber. Then he crawled down the narrow fuselage to his position in the tail gunner's turret. The plexiglass bubble where he rode was so small he had to leave his parachute on the rack in the fuselage. He wore his harness.

The full moon was just rising as the first wave of bombers rolled down the runway and off toward Berlin. The tail gunner's turret is a lonesome spot on a bomber. The gunner is separated from the rest of the crew by the long, narrow fuselage. But Alkemade was used to this position. He tried to doze on the long flight to Berlin.

It was after midnight, and Berlin was blacked out when the first bombers droned in at 21,000 feet. The first ones dropped marker bombs to light up the target area. Within minutes searchlights were stabbing the sky and antiaircraft guns had set up a chatter. The night fighters of the *Luftwaffe* scurried aloft to search out the bombers. But the Lancaster dropped its bombs and circled to head for home.

The bomber was lighter now, and they should make better time on the return flight. Alkemade was just beginning to feel good about this trip, when the Lancaster shook with a series of explosions. A cannon shell grazed and shattered the plexiglass bubble that housed the tail gunner. Alkemade found himself staring into icy space. Then he saw the shadowy form of the black Junkers 88 on their tail. The sergeant aimed his Browning and fired point-blank at the Junkers. Its port engine exploded, and the plane fell toward the earth in flames.

The Lancaster was on fire. Flaming gasoline streamed past the open tail gunner's turret. The voice of the captain came over the intercom. "I can't hold her much longer, boys. You'll have to jump. Bail out! Bail out!"

Alkemade would have to get his parachute from the fuselage. He opened the door. Flames seared his face. Alkemade pulled his leather helmet down as low as possible and shielded his face with his arms. His only hope was to get through those flames to his parachute. Then he saw that his canopy was on fire. As he watched in horror, it turned black and disintegrated. There was no other parachute.

Flight Sergeant Alkemade knew he was going to die. The flames were searing his face and hands. The pain was unbearable. He tumbled out backward into space.

The cool air was soothing on Alkemade's burned face. He felt calm and peaceful as he fell over and over from 18,000 feet up. If this is dying, he thought as he floated through the air, it isn't so bad after all.

When Alkemade came to, he was bitterly cold. I'm dead, he thought. But if this is death, it isn't at all what I expected. Alkemade hurt all over and ached from the cold.

He reached into his pocket and found some matches. Lighting one, he looked around. He seemed to be in a snowbank. Above him, he could see the interlaced branches of fir trees. Trees were thick all around him. He was in a forest. Slowly Alkemade came to the conclusion that he had fallen 18,000 feet, but was still alive. Carefully he moved each part of his body, trying to find out how badly he was injured. He decided that his face, hands, and legs were burned. His knee was twisted, his back was strained, and he had numerous cuts. But he was in pretty good shape. If he stayed in this snowbank much longer, he would freeze. In the fall, he had somehow lost both boots, and his clothes were in shreds. Alkemade began to yell for help.

Some farm people found the flyer and took him to a farmhouse. The Gestapo was called, and policemen hauled Alkemade off to the hospital to be treated. After he was patched up, they began to question him.

"Where is your parachute?"

"It burned up on the airplane. I jumped without one."

"You lie, Englishman. Where did you bury it?"

For the next three weeks Alkemade was questioned. When he said he jumped without a parachute, he was beaten. His life became a nightmare. Then, one night while lying sleepless, the answer came to him. He could prove his story.

Before sending him off to the prisoner-of-war camp, the Germans questioned Alkemade again. This time the questioner was Lieutenant Feidal of the *Luftwaffe*. He spoke English fluently.

"Where is your parachute?" he began.

"I jumped without one."

Alkemade could see the rising anger in the lieutenant's

face. He added quickly, "If you will send for the harness I was wearing when I was picked up, I can prove my story."

The harness was sent for, and Alkemade put it on. He showed the lieutenant that the hooks and lift webs were still tied down with thread. Any airman would know that these threads would break when the parachute was opened.

Lieutenant Feidal looked incredulous. "Let me see that," he said.

After this, Alkemade was a hero to the Germans. He had jumped 18,000 feet without a parachute and survived. They wrote out an affidavit to the effect that his story had been investigated and found to be true.

Maybe this story doesn't belong in a chapter on parachute jumping. But the record shows that Alkemade made the greatest no-parachute jump of all time. No one, so far, has even attempted to equal it.

Let's go back to the start of World War II and see how parachutes were used then. By this time airmen from all major countries were using parachutes. The principal use was, of course, to help pilots escape from disabled aircraft. But new uses were quickly found. As soon as war was declared, Hitler sent night flights to drop sea mines, attached to parachutes, in Britain's harbors and estuaries. The parachutes let the mines down gently so that they wouldn't blow up on impact. Land mines were also dropped by parachute over England. When a bomb is dropped from an airplane, it is often buried too deep to do much damage. If attached to a parachute, it explodes on the surface and causes more damage.

In World War II, huge airborne armies came into use for the first time. Sometimes there was no way to supply these troops except by air. This was the case in Burma. Allied troops there were surrounded by jungles and Japanese troops. All supplies had to be parachuted in. Vast numbers of parachutes were necessary to make these supply drops. Silk was used for personnel parachutes before World War

II. But the Allies' supply of silk was cut off by the Japanese. A replacement had to be found in a hurry. The new synthetic fabric, nylon, seemed to be the answer. Nylon, though, was in short supply. Parachutes for dropping supplies were made out of cotton or jute. By the end of the war Germany was making them out of paper.

In World War I, parachutes were used to drop spies and saboteurs behind enemy lines. This practice continued during World War II. The Germans added a new twist. Three men and their weapons were shut inside a container 9 feet long and 6 feet in diameter. Four parachutes were used to float it gently down to earth. After the saboteurs had finished their work, they returned and locked themselves inside the container. A low-flying aircraft then hooked them aloft without landing.

Soon after the close of World War I, General Billy Mitchell declared that parachute troops would play a part in the next war. He began to experiment with airborne troops in the early 1920s. In 1928, General Mitchell demonstrated his concept of paratroopers at Kelly Field, Texas, before military observers. Six infantrymen parachuted down with their equipment. Within three minutes they had set up machine guns and were ready to fight. This demonstration did not impress the officers of the U.S. Army. Observers from Germany and Russia were also present. They were impressed.

Germany and Russia began to train squadrons of parachute troops. At the opening of World War II, in the winter of 1939–40, Russia dropped paratroopers behind the Finnish lines. These men were then equipped with machine guns, ammunition, and supplies from the air. Germany used paratroopers for the first time against Norway. Later, they were used against the Netherlands and Belgium. Airborne troops in great numbers were dropped in the Battle of Crete. Thousands of German paratroopers succeeded in capturing the island. But Hitler decided that the price was too high. Destroyed in that battle were 4,000 German troops and 170 aircraft. Never again did Hitler launch a full-scale airborne attack.

The Allies were slower in seeing the value of paratroops. Eventually, though, a complete army of sky soldiers was formed. Toward the end of the war, Allied paratroops spearheaded the invasion of Normandy. Paratroopers were used in the South Pacific. Two thousand of them jumped from 500 feet to recapture Corregidor. At the infamous prison camp at Los Banos, 125 paratroopers landed to free 2,147 sick and wounded prisoners. Paratroopers in the U.S. Army were all volunteers from other branches of the services.

Help for the wounded often came by parachute. Paramedics were landed to help the wounded. In Britain some sincere men refused to engage in combat because of religious beliefs. These men were assigned a much tougher task than serving on the front line. The British Medical Corps was largely made up of noncombatants. The men landed behind enemy lines to administer first aid to the wounded. They were each issued a revolver for protection of themselves and the wounded. Most refused to wear one and landed on D-day unarmed. Field ambulances and medical supplies were parachuted in with them. Usually the group included at least one surgeon. The paramedics landed and set up a field surgery and dressing station. Often the surgeon operated within sound of enemy gunfire.

During World War II, pilots ran into a new problem. High-performance military aircraft came into general use. Before the war, the low speeds of airplanes presented no obstacle to a jumper. But at high speed, the pilot was often pressed back into the cockpit and couldn't bail out. Many of the pilots who were able to get out were injured when thrown against the airplane. A survey in 1943 showed that 12½ percent of emergency parachute jumps were fatal. Of the men who survived, 45½ percent were injured. Most of these injuries resulted from colliding with some part of the airplane. Some device was needed to catapult the pilot away from the disabled aircraft.

The Germans had been working on an ejection seat since 1939. By 1944, these seats were standard equipment on their Messerschmitt airplanes. Over sixty seat ejections were made in the first year of their use.

But the Germans and the Allies weren't exchanging ideas. The Allies had to come up with their own design. Unfortunately, it didn't come in time to help World War II fighter pilots. Sweden installed ejection seats on their fighters in 1945. Britain successfully tested the Martin-Baker ejection seat that same year. The United States adopted the British-designed ejection seat soon after.

The problem of escaping from a high-speed airplane was not solved for all time when ejection seats were designed for World War II fighter planes. Each time a solution was found, a new and faster airplane was developed. The Department of Defense Joint Parachute Test Facility at El Centro, California, continually evaluates new escape systems. Today, rockets are used to blast the pilot out of the cockpit. On these escapes, ninety-five of every one hundred ejections are successful.

PRESENT AND FUTURE USE OF PARACHUTES

The parachute is the best known and most reliable device for lowering something to the ground from a high altitude. The canopy provides enough drag so that the object will descend slowly, and it is less expensive to use than a helicopter. New uses for parachutes are being found all the time.

Parachutes were first used for lowering heavy loads in 1921. During World War II, the military used them to land everything from tanks to field hospitals. Since then, civilians have put them to work to land equally heavy equipment. Parachutes used for heavy loads are different from those used for personnel. They are composed of concentric rings of fabric with openings to permit more air to flow through. This type of parachute is highly stable and suitable for supporting heavy loads. Sometimes a cluster of parachutes is used.

Today parachutes are used for many commercial purposes. The American Telephone and Telegraph Company uses parachutes to lower repeaters to a predetermined depth in the ocean. These devices, which help boost telephone messages, must be installed every twenty-five miles.

As the distance a helicopter can fly is limited, parachutes are often the only way to deliver needed materials to inaccessible areas. Heavy oil-surveying and construction equipment often arrives at the Arctic sites by air. Mining equipment has been parachuted into the jungle. One of these loads was 22 tons of steel plate, dropped with a cluster of six parachutes.

Parachutes are used to gather information about weather conditions in the stratosphere. This is the region which extends from about eleven to thirty miles above the earth. An 8-foot rocket is fired to an average of forty-five miles above the earth. At the highest point a small explosive charge forces off the nose cone and pulls the 15-foot parachute out of the container. A sensor and a transmitter are attached to the parachute. The sensor is sensitive to temperature changes, and this information is transmitted back to the meteorological base. Since alternate gores on the parachute are coated with a silverized copper finish, the parachute can be tracked by radar. From its drift, wind direction and velocity can be calculated.

Could a parachute be used to lower a disabled airplane safely? The answer is yes. This was first done with a small airplane in 1927. After Major Hoffman and his staff solved the problem of a safe parachute for people, they decided to develop a parachute that could land a disabled airplane safely. In 1927, R. Carl Oelze demonstrated a 50-foot chute he had developed. At 3,000 feet he turned off the plane's engine and opened a parachute attached to the top wing. The parachute took over and lowered the Curtiss biplane safely.

In April 1929, Colonel Roscoe Turner demonstrated the use of a parachute to land a powerless aircraft safely. At 5,000 feet, Turner cut the switch on his Thunderbird biplane. A 60-foot parachute opened and brought the airplane to earth.

Other tests followed the first two. Some were successful; some were failures. But the idea never caught on. There were problems. A parachute large enough to lower a modern commercial airplane couldn't be packed into the fuselage. The U.S. Air Force researchers turned their attention to the problem. They came up with a plan in which separate parachutes would be attached to different sections of the aircraft. In an emergency, the pilot would pull a handle that would detonate small charges of explosives. These would slice the aircraft into separate segments, which could then be lowered by individual parachutes. The idea was never tested.

The idea of individual parachutes for passengers on large commercial airplanes has often been discussed. This idea has been discouraged by the airlines. There are many arguments against such a plan. The airlines feel that furnishing parachutes would frighten passengers. In addition, most accidents occur while the airplane is landing or taking off. Parachutes would be useless then. The high altitude at which modern commercial planes fly also presents a problem. Each passenger would have to be supplied with oxygen for the jump. There will probably be no parachutes on commercial airlines.

There seems to be an appalling lack of interest in aircraft safety by those who should be most concerned. Almost no civilian pilots or passengers on small aircraft wear parachutes. Even pilots in the military receive no instructions in jumping. If they make a jump, it is during an emergency. There have been many fatal accidents because, in the excitement of the first bailout, the pilot did the wrong thing.

Parachutes are used on the ground today to slow rapidly moving vehicles. Many supersonic airplanes are equipped with parachutes to enable them to land on short runways. Commercial airplanes, such as the *Concorde* and the *Caravelle,* are equipped with parachutes. They are also used on fighter planes—both land based and carrier based. High-speed racing automobiles, such as those used in drag races and to establish speed records, depend on the braking action of parachutes.

Today, personnel parachutes are made of nylon and are exceptionally strong. As many as twenty-eight different

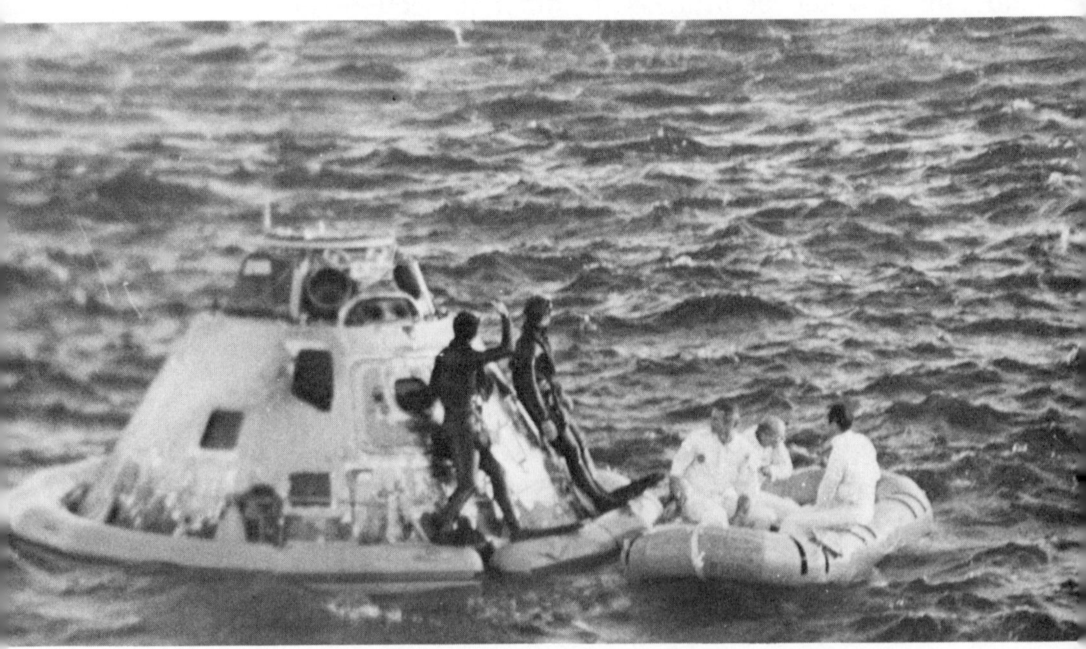

Navy frogmen have been dropped to aid astronauts

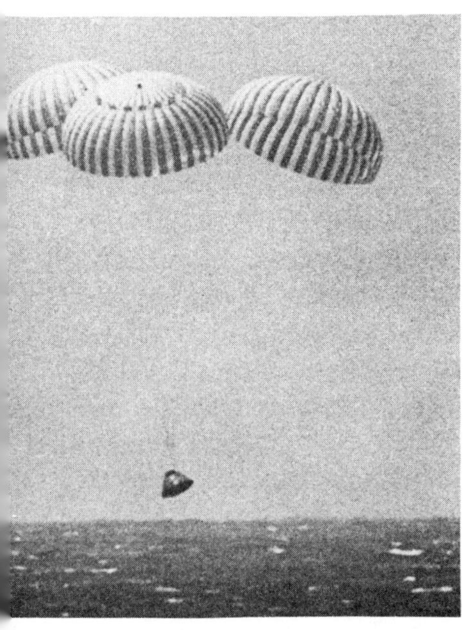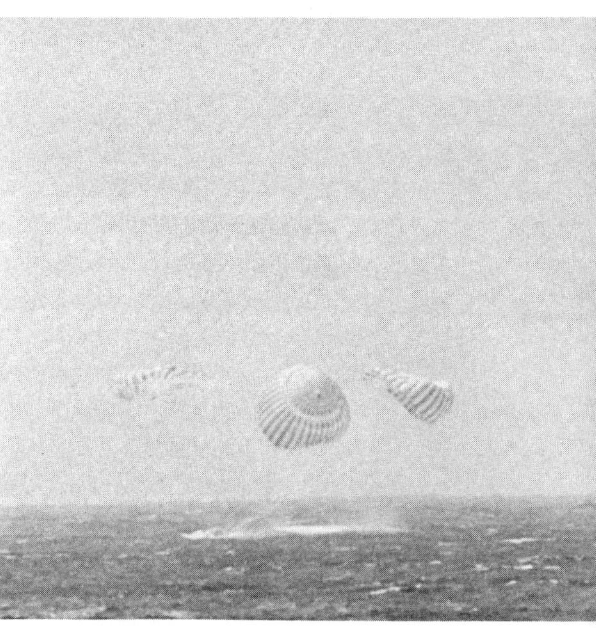

Landing of the Apollo 12 spacecraft

gores or sections are used in each one. A tear in one section does not spread to the rest of the canopy. Let's look at some of the new uses for these people-carrying parachutes.

As we have seen, paramedics were first dropped from airplanes in World War II. This practice continued after the close of the war. Today, paramedics and pararescue teams are dropped into isolated areas whenever help is needed. After a disaster, such as an earthquake or a flood, this may be the only way to help victims. Doctors, nurses, and medical assistants can be dropped by parachute. Lifeboats can be dropped after a disaster at sea.

Parascuba diving is one of the newest uses for the parachute. A diver, complete with rubber suit, swim fins, and aqualung, can be parachuted down when necessary. One mining company used parascuba divers to map underwater gold deposits. Some divers have been used to locate sunken ships. The Armed Forces use parascuba divers. Commando type of activities can be carried out by divers who descend silently from the sky and complete their missions in the

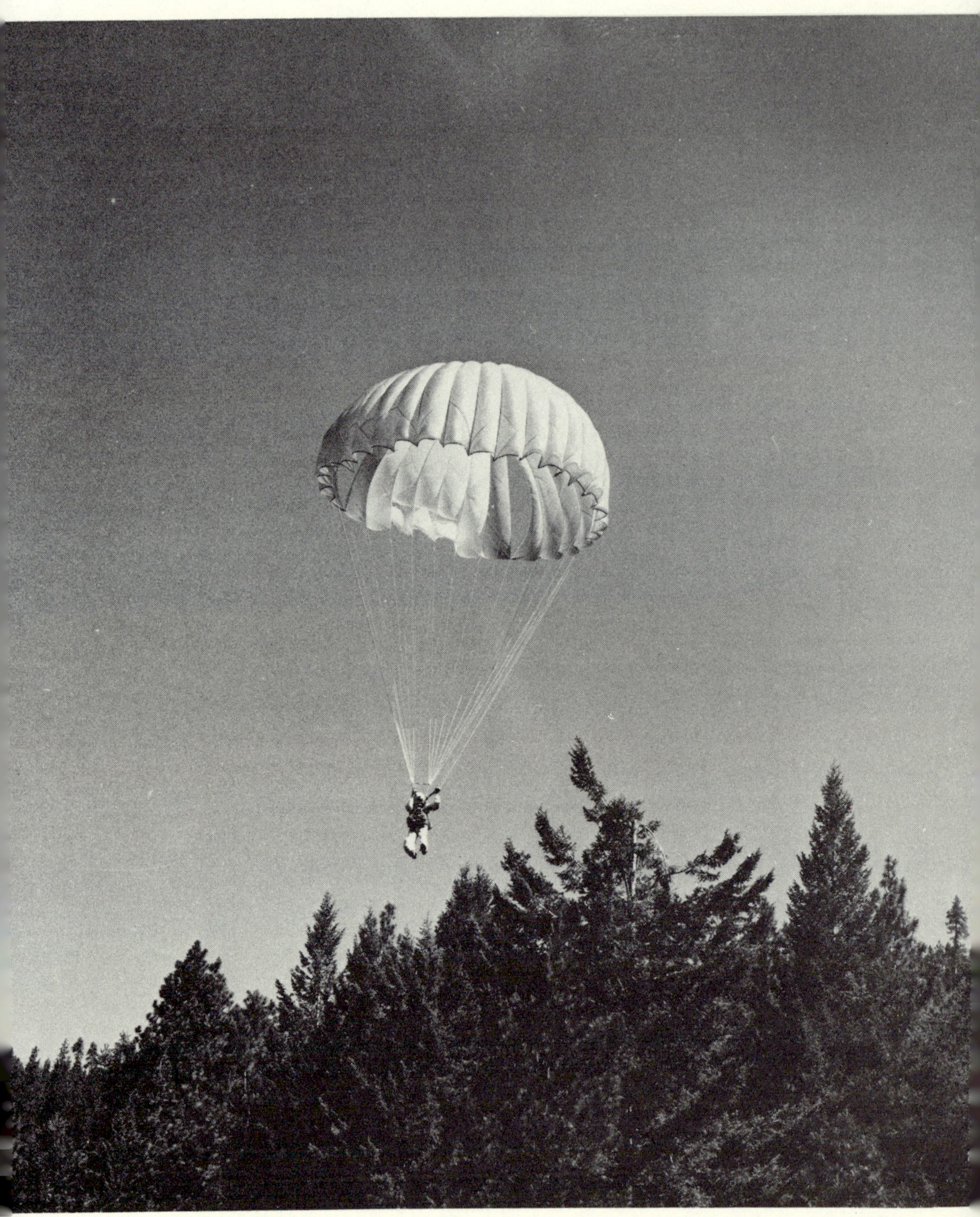

dark. Have you ever watched the recovery of a space capsule from the ocean? Parascuba divers are dropped either by parachute or from low-flying helicopters to stabilize the capsule and assist the astronauts.

Smoke jumpers have been used since 1940 by the Forest Service to control fires in the Western mountains. A highly maneuverable chute was needed to enable the jumpers to land safely in the rugged forested areas. The parachute now used was adapted from one used by paratroopers. Today, when there is a forest fire, the smoke jumper is the first line of defense.

The National Geographic Society used parachutes to land explorers in an inaccessible area of Peru. Their supplies also arrived by chutes. After completing the mission, the four explorers built a balsa raft and floated down out of the Andes Mountains.

Photographers sometimes use parachutes to enable them to snap otherwise unattainable pictures. News and television cameramen have taken to parachutes to get the photographs they want.

Both Russian and American astronauts have made the final leg of their descent from space by parachute. The Russians have landed all their astronauts on the ground. Yuri Gagarin, who was the world's first cosmonaut in 1961, landed in a capsule suspended from a parachute. In all other Russian space missions, the airman was shot from the capsule by a rocket-powered ejection seat. Then the parachute opened and the astronaut floated back to earth. One Russian astronaut, Colonel Vladimir Komarov, was killed on one of these landings when his parachute lines became entangled four miles above the earth.

The United States has chosen to land the capsules used for the Mercury, Gemini, and Apollo shots in the ocean. Because of the cushioning effect of the water, a smaller parachute can be used. The 1971 mission of Apollo 15 almost ended in disaster. The capsule was equipped with three parachutes, but only two deployed. The three astronauts were warned, "Be prepared for a hard impact." But the landing contained a built-in margin of safety. Two parachutes were enough for a safe, if rather fast, reentry.

Rocket-powered ejection seats are built into all space capsules. If there should be a mishap on the launching pad, the seat would be shot about 900 feet into the air. Then the parachute would open and bring the astronaut safely back to earth.

Parachutes play a part in the exploration of the planets. Soviet scientists used a parachute to land a spacecraft, *Venera 4,* on Venus. As the temperature of this planet is 540 degrees Fahrenheit, a special parachute was built to withstand the heat.

On July 20, 1976, NASA landed the spacecraft *Viking I* on Mars. When the entry speed of the lander had slowed to 600 miles per hour, a parachute was deployed. After the lander settled softly to the surface of Mars, the parachute was released.

But the big growth in the use of parachutes today is because people have found that parachute jumping is fun. Every weekend thousands of jumpers joyfully launch themselves into space. We will take a look at what they are doing in the next chapter on sport parachuting and skydiving.

8. SKYDIVING

WHY JUMP?

The small airplane circled high overhead. Heads bent back and faces were turned to the sky as people watched. Then a speck appeared under the plane. Slowly it turned in the air, looking like a paper doll dropped from a window. The spectators began to shift their feet and murmur. When would the chute open? Then a long ribbon trailed out behind the figure. A brilliant-colored canopy bloomed in the sky. There was an audible sigh of relief from the crowd. The fearful plunge through space had been halted. They watched as the jumper tugged at the risers to guide himself into a perfect spot landing. Another day of skydiving was under way.

What is skydiving? Sport parachuting is any jump made with a parachute for fun. The term "skydiving" is applied to jumps with a long free fall.

Sport jumping appeared long before skydiving. But today skydiving is one of the fastest-growing sports in the United States. An average of over four thousand jumps are made for pleasure every day. Most sport parachutists have switched to skydiving. But what enjoyment is there in risking life by throwing oneself into empty space with only a piece of fabric to bring one safely down to earth?

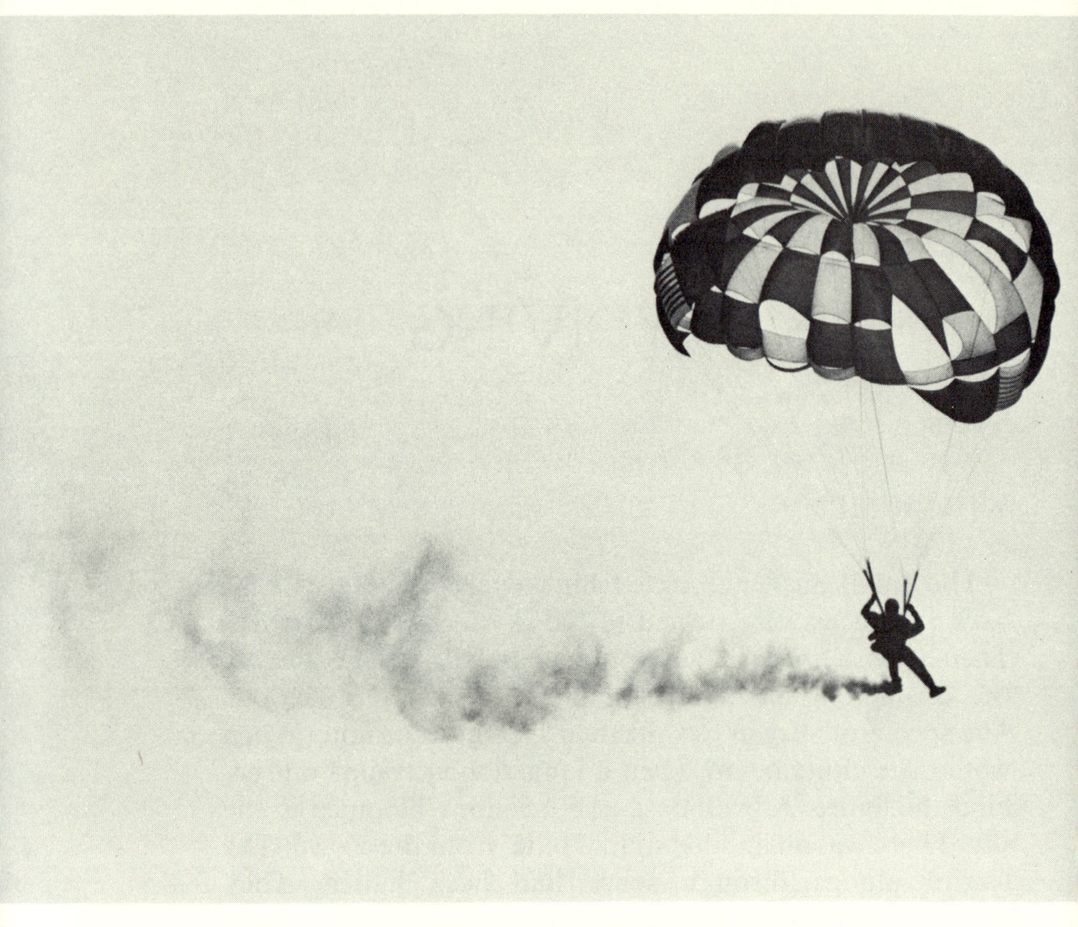

*Some parachutists jump for entertainment, like
the Navy jumper trailing colored smoke*

If you ask a skydiver this question, he or she will talk
about the thrill of using one's own skills to cheat death.
This is the same thrill shared by race car drivers and those
who participate in other dangerous sports. Dedicated skydivers talk about the personal challenge of jumping. Courage and ability to think clearly under stress are needed for
each jump. It is an adventure that only a few have the skill
and opportunity to share.

At first, parachute jumps were made to entertain crowds.

Then the emphasis shifted to the use of parachutes for safety. Today, although the parachute is still used as a safety device, the emphasis is back again on parachuting for fun. Where and when did sport parachuting and skydiving get their start?

The Pulitzer Air Races were held in Philadelphia in 1926. At these races it was customary to have a few parachute jumps to entertain the crowd. Joe Crane, organizer of the National Parachute Jumpers Association (NPJA), suggested that a spot-landing contest be held. The jumpers try to land on or near a target. Later, Crane organized spot-landing contests for other air races. These exhibitions were watched with interest. But sport parachuting did not catch on in the United States at that time. Membership in the NPJA barely reached two hundred by World War II.

Sport parachuting in Europe became popular long before it did in the United States. As we have seen, Russia and Germany began to train parachute troops between the two world wars. This led to an interest in sport parachuting in those countries. By 1930, parachuting had become a mass pastime in the Soviet Union. Schools were set up to train parachutists. To reduce the cost, jumps were often made from special tall towers. Entire Russian families would spend the afternoon tower jumping. By 1936, Russia had over fifteen hundred jumping towers and over one hundred jumping schools. Parachute jumping also became very popular in Germany.

During World War II, many men from the United States were trained as paratroopers. After the war many of them wanted to continue jumping as a sport. Small groups of enthusiasts, mostly ex-paratroopers, began organizing jumping clubs.

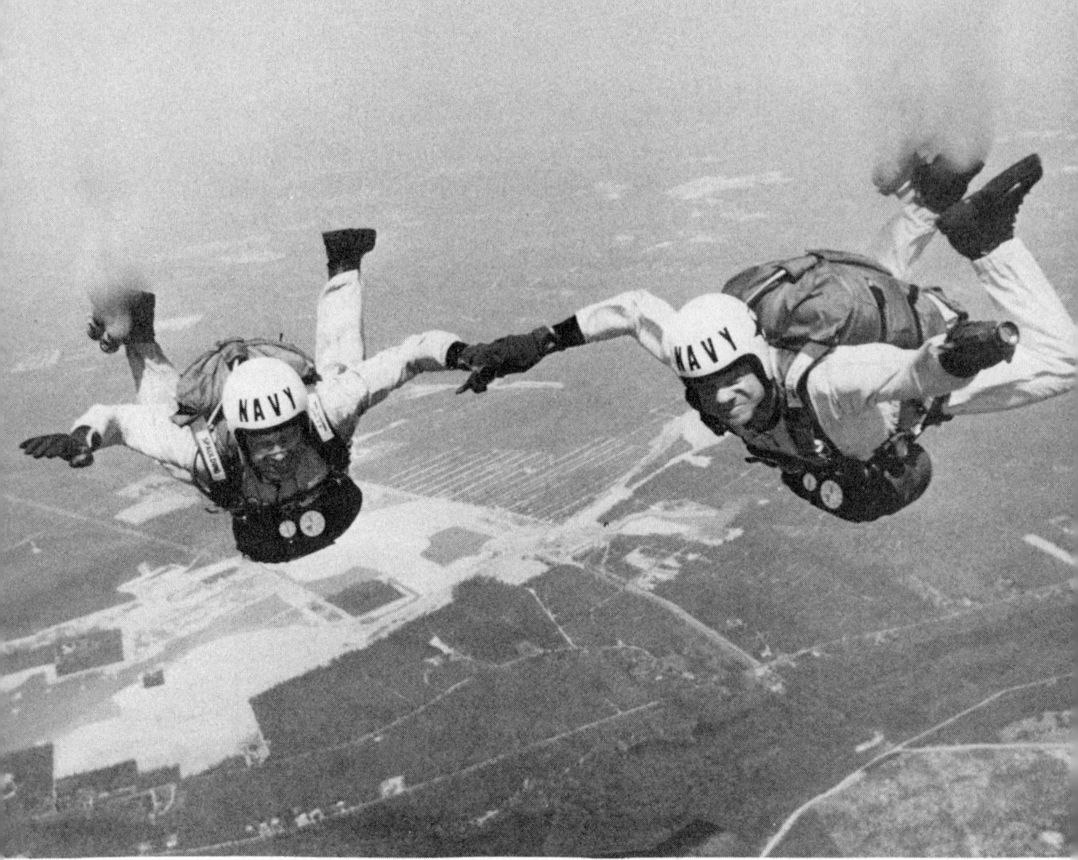

*Group jumping is difficult and body contact
dangerous*

SKYDIVING—U.S.A.

Sput—sput—sput—sput—sput! Jacques André Istel
looked anxiously at the instrument panel. He couldn't be
out of gas. No, something else was wrong with the plane.
But no gas was getting through to the engine—of that he
was sure. Now the engine died completely. Jacques worked
frantically trying to get it started again. No luck. The
twenty-year-old graduate of Princeton stared down at the
Illinois countryside. Was his short life over so soon? Recent
events flashed through his mind. Jacques had just learned
to fly. In order to get an airplane of his own, he had gone

122

to Vancouver, British Columbia, and bought this surplus war plane. It had seemed a bargain at $600. But now the engine on his bargain has stopped and there was no place to land. Why hadn't he worn a parachute?

Then Jacques Istel saw the potato field. It wasn't much, but it seemed to be the best place to try for an emergency landing. Jacques brought his new airplane down for a rough but safe landing. This experience shook Jacques up. He realized he had been very close to death. "From now on," he vowed, "I'll wear a parachute." But then he realized he wouldn't know how to jump if he had to. Jacques had never made a parachute jump.

A few days later Jacques Istel went to see Joe Crane. He wanted to learn how to make a parachute jump. His first

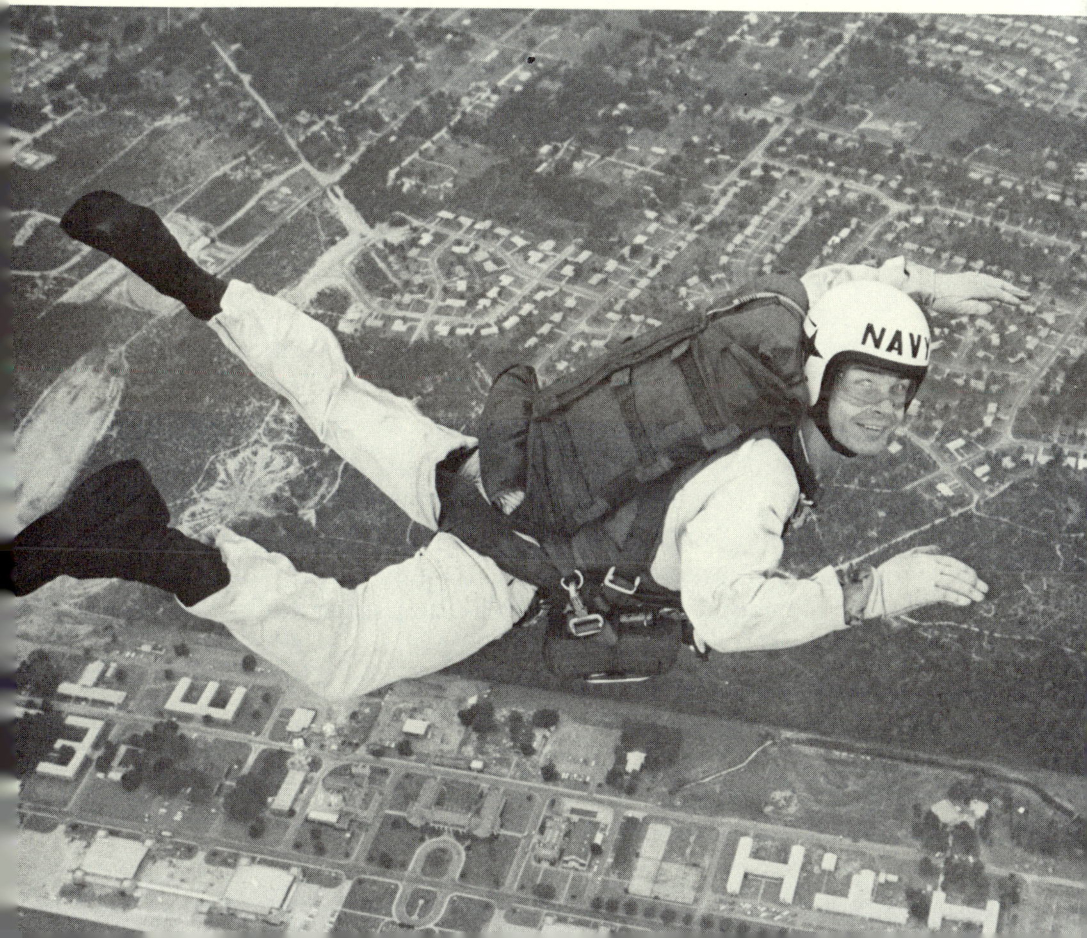

The spread-eagle position keeps the body from tumbling

jump wasn't a big success. He nearly landed on top of another airplane. But after that, his jumping improved, and he became enthusiastic about this new sport. Later, during the Korean War, Istel served with the U.S. Marines as a paratrooper. He became Captain Istel.

In 1956, the Third International Parachuting Championship was to be held in Moscow. At this time parachuting was dominated by Europeans—especially those behind the Iron Curtain. The United States had never sent a jumping team to the championships. In 1954, one jumper, Fred Mason, had gone to France alone to represent the United States. Some members of the NPJA felt the United States should organize and send a team to this championship. But there was one serious problem. Two of the events would be in skydiving. No one in the United States knew how to skydive.

Captain Jacques Istel went to France to learn free-fall techniques from Sam Chasak, France's national parachuting champion. Chasak taught Istel the rudiments of skydiving and how to stabilize and maneuver his body during free fall. Istel learned how to perform turns, loops, and rolls while falling.

Back in the United States, Jacques Istel and Joe Crane invited fifty of the best parachute jumpers to meet to form a parachuting team. They chose six to participate. These six jumpers watched while Istel went up to demonstrate how to maneuver during free fall. All were skeptical of this new stunt. They had all been jumping much longer than had Istel. But the veteran jumpers watched in astonishment while Istel executed graceful figure eights while falling. All were wildly enthusiastic about this new method of jumping.

For six weeks the newly formed team worked from dawn to dusk, practicing and learning all Istel could teach them. The team went to Moscow as the United States Parachuting Team. The Americans didn't come in first, but they did very well.

124

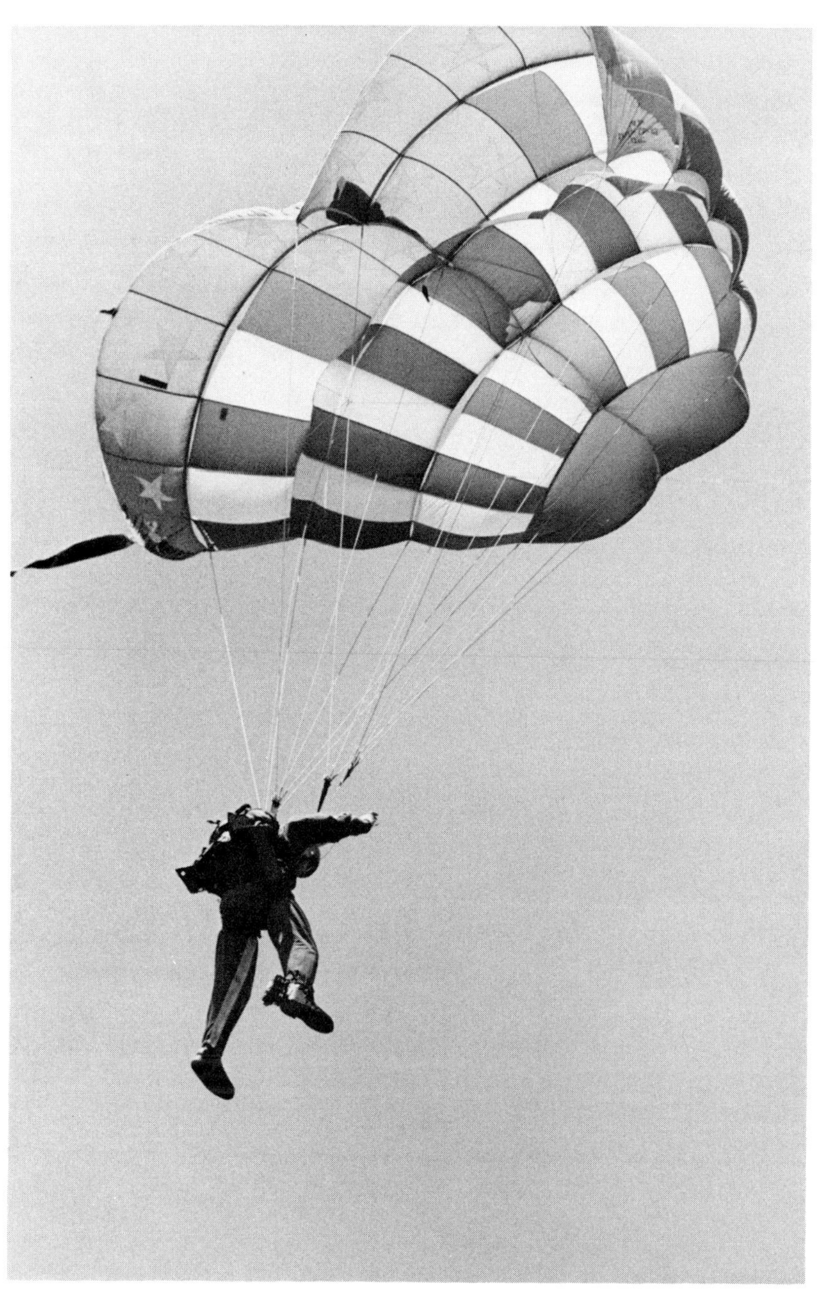

A skydiving entertainer knows when he must pull the rip cord

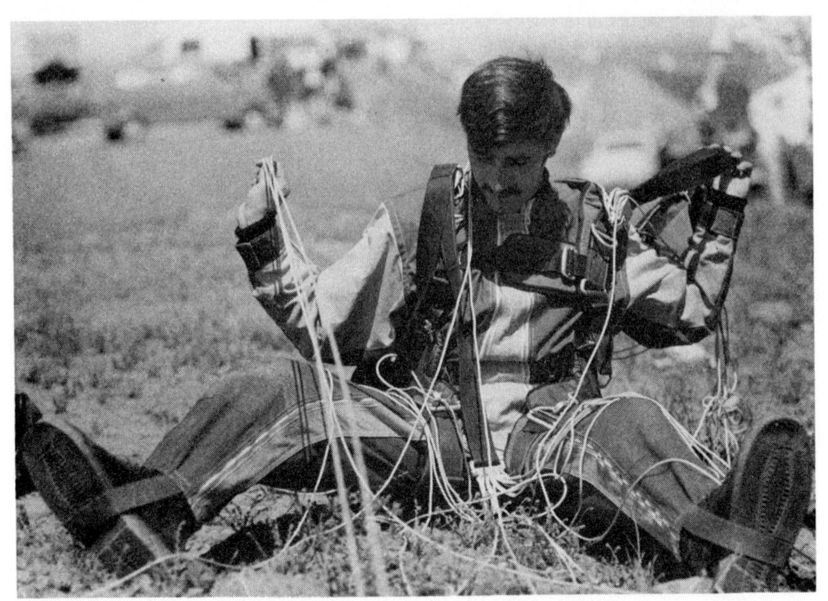

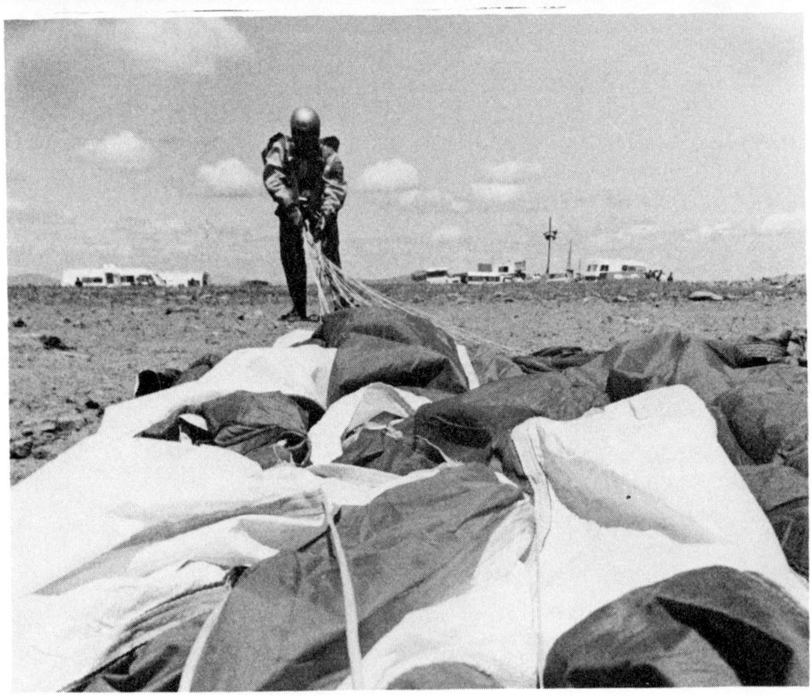

After landing, he untangles himself and straightens the guidelines on his chute

126

After a few skydiving exhibitions in the United States, the sport caught on. Soon American jumpers were amazing the rest of the world with their skill. Today there are many parachuting clubs and jumping teams in the United States.

Parachute competitions and exhibitions are now held in every state. Skydivers have come up with new stunts. The most exciting and dangerous are those involving several people. The baton pass is very popular. Two jumpers leave the airplane a short time apart, one carrying a baton. During free fall, the two jumpers try to maneuver their bodies so the baton can be passed from one to the other. Since little communication is possible during a jump, careful planning is necessary.

During jumping competitions, teams and individuals compete for points on style and landing accuracy. In judging style, no attention is paid to where the jumper lands. In judging accuracy, team members are judged by how close they land to the center of a target marked out on the ground.

Group jumping is more difficult and dangerous. There is always the chance of parachute lines becoming entangled. Teams, such as the Army's Golden Knights from Fort Bragg, North Carolina, give exhibitions. They maneuver themselves into circles and other formations during free fall. The Golden Knights have won many world championships. Part of their success is due to a remarkable parachute that was developed especially for their use. It has thirty-six slots and vents to give maximum maneuverability and lift. It actually flies. The Knights are showmen. Each one has a bracket on the side of his boot to hold a smoke grenade. During their dives, they are followed by red, green, yellow, and purple smoke trails. There are always oohs and aahs from the spectators when the Golden Knights perform.

During a free fall, the slightest movement of an arm or leg changes the position of the body. To some extent it also influences the speed and direction of the descent. Several basic stable positions are used. Most are variations of the spread-eagle position, with arms and legs held out and slightly back.

A wrist altimeter and a stopwatch are worn and used on all jumps. French skydivers have buzzers inside their helmets that sound when it is time to pull the rip cord. It is easy to misjudge altitude. Most fatal accidents occur when the jumper fails to open the parachute in time. A skydiver can become so engrossed in the thrill of a free fall that he or she forgets to pull the rip cord until too late. During free fall the jumper reaches a velocity of over 120 miles an hour, but there is no feeling of speed. There is just the wind rushing by your body and tugging at your clothes.

One of the biggest dangers in skydiving is overconfidence and the carelessness it brings. During the first few jumps, skydivers are very careful. Equipment and procedure are checked. After a few successful jumps, there is a tendency to forget that one's life hangs by a thin thread. Jumpers begin to think nothing can happen to them. Each succeeding jump should be approached with the same caution as the first.

It would be impossible and dangerous to try to learn parachuting from a book. Read all you like about the sport. But if you are really interested in getting into parachute jumping, write to the U.S. Parachute Association, Suite 444, 806 15th Street, N.W., Washington, D.C. 20005, for more information. They will send you a booklet about parachuting schools and clubs. The sport should only be undertaken with good equipment and a skilled instructor.

9. PARASAILING

IT'S EASY TO TRY

What blooms like a huge tropical flower over almost any crowded beach today? What is the center of attention for all the sun lovers tanning on the sand? What new experience are all the young people clamoring to try? It is parasailing—the parachute that rises and flies.

The parasail is the safest and least expensive way to try parachuting. Customers are taken up for a five- or ten-minute ride. The canopy looks much like that of any parachute, except that there are more vents or slots to provide lift. Before there can be lift, there must be forward motion. This is provided by a speedboat.

Suppose you have paid your money, and it is your turn to fly with the parasail. What happens? You will probably be quite nervous as you are helped into a harness and buckled up. You grasp the straps while sitting on a wide leather or plastic strap. Your legs just dangle. Now the assistants stand on each side of the canopy and hold it out so the cloth will scoop air on takeoff. When all is ready, they signal the speedboat driver and assistant, who are waiting just off the beach. The boat gives a *r-r-r-r-o-o-o-o-o-o-o-m-m-m-m-m-m* and surges forward. You are tugged ahead and you begin to run. But after a few steps, you find yourself

129

running in empty air. You feel rather silly and stop. Your feet skim just out of reach of the water. You are off!

Now that you are in the air, you realize that your heart is beating fast and your hands are wet with perspiration. But that is all behind you. You feel exhilarated and at peace. The water and swimmers recede rapidly beneath you. Now you can look around. You can see over the buildings lining the beach and see the automobiles on the street and the people on the sidewalk. You shout at them, "Look at me! I'm flying!"

All of a sudden you realize you are singing as loud as possible. Don't be alarmed. Most parasailers feel like singing. The wind blows your hair. But, other than that, you have no feeling of speed. It is quite comfortable up here under the big colorful canopy. Now the speedboat begins to make a big half circle. Your parasail follows around too. You realize that your ride will soon be over.

Soon you are closer to the people on the beach. Every face is turned up, watching you. You are the center of attention. You feel like a celebrity and wave at them.

The faces are getting larger. You must be sinking. Yes, the speedboat is going slower. Now you see the takeoff place just ahead. The motor boat slows until it almost stops. Without the forward pull, the parachute starts descending. The attendants' arms reach up to help you, and your feet touch the ground.

Quickly the harness is unbuckled. Someone else is waiting to take your place. You stumble as you turn to walk away. Your legs have to get used to the ground again. Already there is one thought in the back of your mind. I must find the money to take another ride.

In the early 1970s, the first parasails appeared on the beaches. Now they are found on most busy seacoasts. Where and when did they get their start? Believe it or not, it was during World War I.

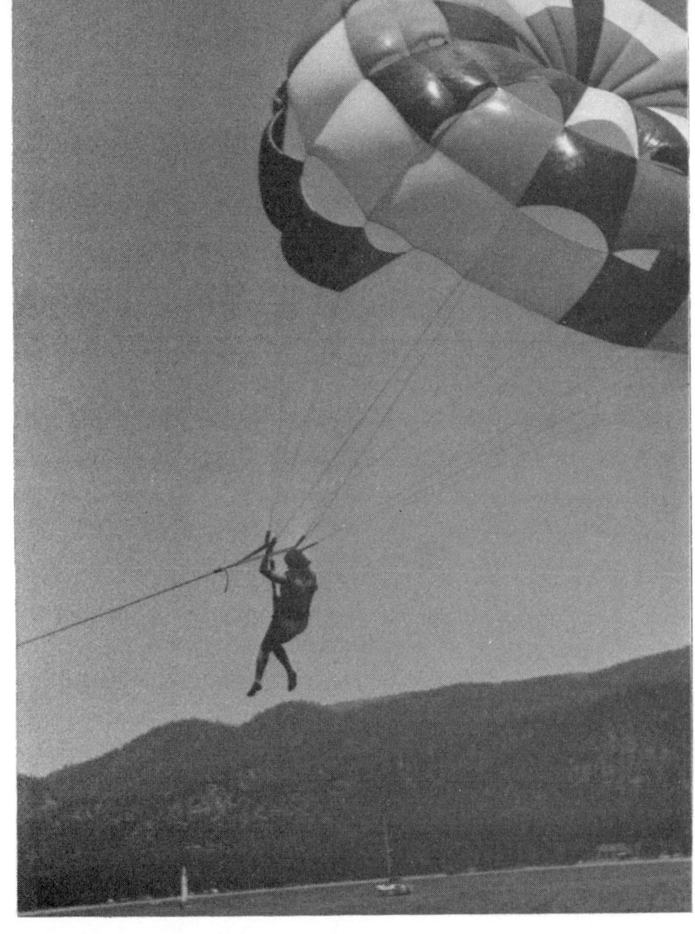

Parasailing is fun!

THE START

In 1918, a German U-boat rose slowly to the surface of the North Atlantic. Then the periscope was raised for a look around. The waves were choppy and it was misty near the water. For the hundredth time, the U-boat captain wished there were some way to have a look around from high over the boat. It was impossible to see anything at sea level.

When the U-boat captain next came in to his home base, he talked this problem over with those in command. He found that other U-boat captains had voiced the same com-

131

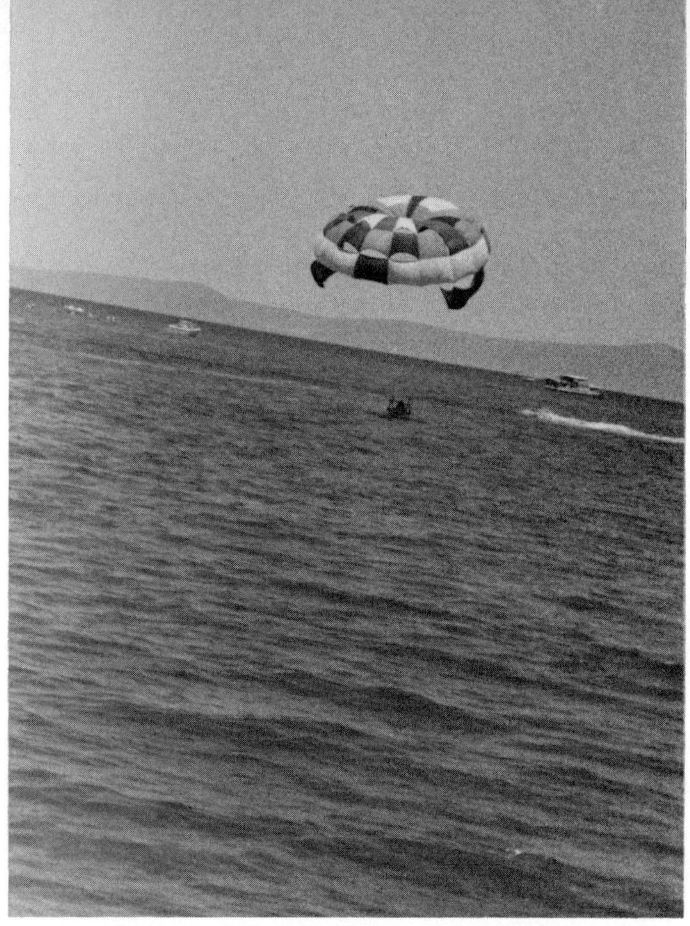

You land on the beach or in the water

plaint. Engineers were working on the problem, and soon they hoped to have a solution.

A few trips later, the U-boat captain was chosen to try out the new secret weapon of the German navy. This was a parachute that had been developed to lift an observer behind the submarine while it was under way on the surface. Its use, though, was limited, as it was often difficult to launch an observer. Soon after this, World War I ended and the project was dropped.

But the idea of a lifting parachute was not totally forgotten. In Britain a multiple airfoil parachute was introduced in 1962. It was used in a sport known as parascending.

132

People were given rides at the beach behind a motor boat and on land behind a car. With some practice a parascender could rise as high as 1,200 feet. A person could travel forward as long as there was forward motion. One girl sailed more than halfway across the English Channel before tiring and coming down. Landing could be made either on land or in the water.

In the United States, the Pioneer Parachute Company also developed a lifting parachute in the 1960s. It was known as the parasail. NASA wanted to give its Apollo astronauts extensive practice in parachuting. In an emergency the astronauts might be required to make a jump. The parasail was used in this training. The astronauts were towed until they had attained a sufficient altitude. Then the parasail was allowed to descend as would any parachute.

For some time after this, little attention was paid to the parasail in the United States. Then someone remembered it. Maybe that person saw it used in Europe. Anyway, some enterprising person in this country bought a parasail, tied it behind a motorboat and went into business giving rides on the beach. The sport caught on at once. From then on it spread and spread. So if you want to try a safe, fun parachute ride, save your money and try the parasail.

PART FOUR / *WIND SPORTS ON WATER, LAND, AND ICE*

10. SAILBOARDS

A NEW SPORT

"What is that funny thing out there?"
"Out where?"
"Out there."
"Oh, that's a surfboard."
"But it has a sail."
"Then it must be a sailboat."
"It doesn't look like any sailboat I've ever seen."

Back in 1966, a strange new craft was sighted one day in the surf off a Southern California beach. All the sunbathers were trying to decide what it was. The surfers were curious too. They got a closer look at it and reported back to the people on the beach. "Someone has put a sail on a surfboard." A sail on a surfboard! What will they think of next?

From time to time one of these crafts—always homemade—appeared off a beach and attracted attention. Hoyle Schweitzer of Southern California saw one of them in 1968. He thought there might be a market for a surfboard with a sail. He began to manufacture them under the name Windsurfer.

Schweitzer sold a few of his new boards in the United States. But they didn't catch on. A visitor from Europe saw and bought a Windsurfer while on a trip here. When he

135

started using it in Europe, the idea caught on. To sailers there, it seemed like the ideal, inexpensive way to enjoy sailing. It didn't require a launching ramp or a trailer, it could be carried on top of a car. It didn't require 10 feet of water under the hull—it would sail in a foot of water. Today there are over three million sailboards in Europe and the sport has returned to the United States.

Sailboarding, or windsurfing, is now growing rapidly in the United States. At least eighty companies here and abroad are now manufacturing the boards. Many schools have been set up to rent and sell sailboards and give lessons.

Let's take a look at a typical sailboard. The first boards were made of fiberglass and were quite heavy. Today most are made of fiberglass-covered foam and are much lighter. Boards vary as to design. Most are 12 feet long and 2 feet in width, and weigh about 45 pounds. There is a mast about 14 feet long and a sail. A small daggerboard keel drops into a slot for greater stability when under way. There is no rudder. The sailboard is steered by the balance and foot-work of the sailer. There is no conventional boom running along the bottom of the sail. The sail is held in place by a wishbone boom which straddles the sail at shoulder height. The entire rig is quickly dismantled when it is to be transported. And, just as quickly, it can be put back together again.

FIRST TIME ON THE WATER

Now how do you sail on a board? Although it looks tricky, sailing on a board is quite easy. It only takes a little instruction and practice before you too are sailing with the wind. Most students master the board in four to six hours. You will learn faster at a school for sailboarding. Lessons begin on dry land, with lectures on wind and sailing technique. Then there is practice on a pivoting simulator, which

136

gives the sensation of sailing the board. After this, it is time to take to the water. First the beginner practices tacking (sailing upwind) and jibbing (sailing downwind). The boom can be operated from either side of the sail.

The beginning windsurfer seems to spend a lot of time falling into the water and crawling back onto the board. Sailboards, though, are remarkably safe. They are so buoyant the U.S. Coast Guard does not require life preservers to be carried. This is the only "boat" exempt from this rule. When you fall into the water, the wet sail acts as a sea anchor and keeps the board from floating away.

There are two requirements for learning how to operate a sailboard. You must weigh at least 85 pounds. It takes strong arms and some weight to pull the sail upright again

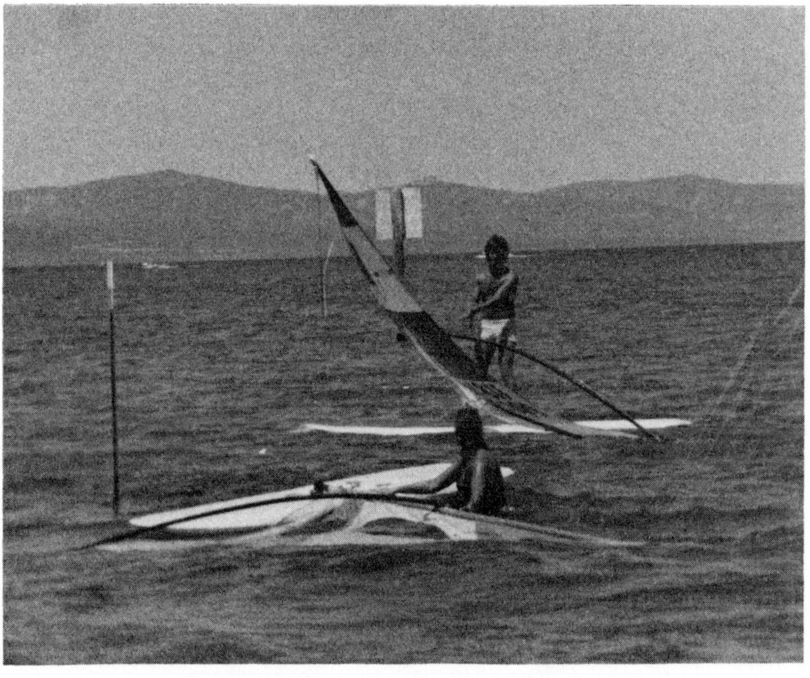

Beginners spend a lot of time falling into the water and crawling back onto the board

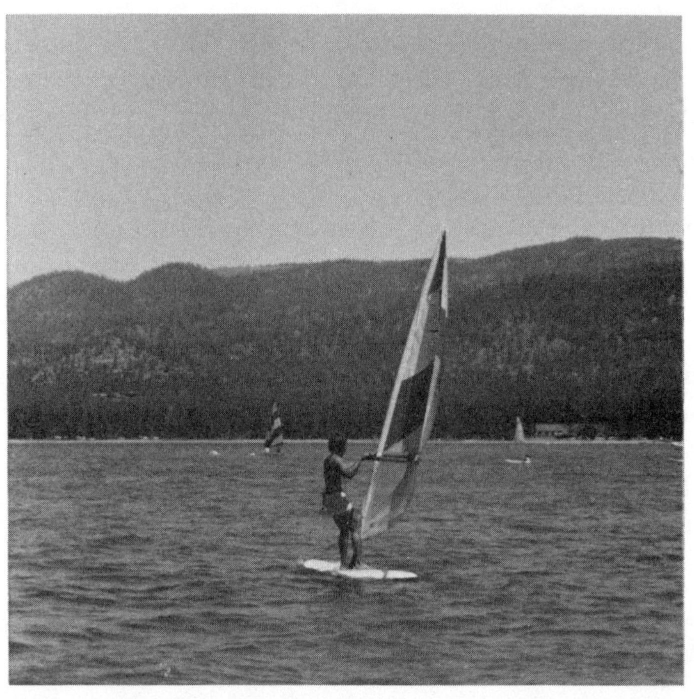

Beginners should only sail in a gentle breeze

after it falls into the water. Also, you must know how to swim. Anyone who has doubts about his or her ability to swim some distance, if necessary, should wear a life jacket. Those under the age of eighteen must have the permission of their parents. Good balance and a little knowledge of sailing will help you to learn the skills faster. If the weather or water is cool, you will be more comfortable in a wet suit.

Beginners sail only in a gentle breeze (under 15 knots). Sometimes lessons have to be rescheduled if it is too windy. Boards can be sailed with only the slightest breeze and are easier to handle then. Skilled windsurfers enjoy the challenge of sailing in a stiff breeze. Speeds of up to 30 miles per hour have been clocked. These speeds make sailboards the fastest of any single-hull sailing craft. Only a large multi-hull racing boat can beat a sailboard.

138

Special boards have been designed for special purposes. Racers and hot-doggers (those who like to do tricks on their boards) prefer a more maneuverable board with a smaller sail. This type of board also performs better in the surf. Extra-stable boards are manufactured for use in the ocean. One rounded Cape Horn, where the ocean is always rough, cruising 137 miles in twenty-four hours.

The boom in windsurfing has just begun. More and more people are discovering this as the purest form of sailing. Sailboarding recently received another boost. A sailboard event will take place in the Olympic games to be held in

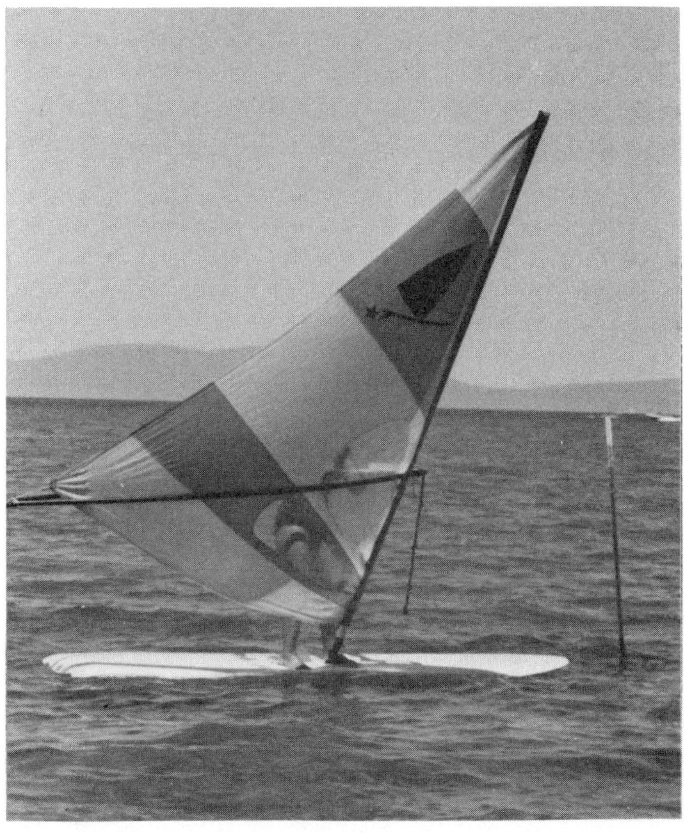

The fastest growing sport

Long Beach, California, in 1984. The International Olympic Committee has officially accepted sailboarding as a new sport.

Dedicated windsurfers will want to join the U.S. Board Sailing Association. The address is Box 206, Oyster Bay, N.Y. 11771. The USBSA sponsors regattas and sets up rules for sailboard races.

11. ICEBOATING

ICEBOATS LONG AGO

Winter had a tight grip on New York State that January day in 1790. For days the temperature had not climbed above zero. At Poughkeepsie, the Hudson River was frozen from bank to bank.

If you had walked down the main street of Poughkeepsie on that long-ago Sunday afternoon, you wouldn't have found many people around. No, they weren't inside huddled by their fireplaces. If you had listened, you could have heard laughter and voices coming from the river.

The frozen river might seem like an unlikely place for a Sunday-afternoon gathering in January. But, in those days, this scene was repeated at every village up and down the river. Everyone was enjoying a clear afternoon on the ice. Men, women, and children were skating. Babies were being pulled on sleds or pushed in baby carriages on runners. Groups stood around the big bonfires on the bank. But there seemed to be some excitement. What were all the people talking about?

"Look at that thing out there on the ice!"

"It's Hans Schmidt. Look what he's made."

"I haven't seen one of those since we left the old country."

"How fast he goes before the wind."

The object of all this attention looked like a wooden box with a sail. It glided over the ice faster than anything anyone had seen travel before.

The Dutch people at Poughkeepsie all recognized Hans Schmidt's strange-looking craft for what it was—an iceboat. Those who were old enough to remember had seen iceboats used on the canals in the Netherlands. Those who had never seen them had heard about them.

Hans Schmidt had built a simple wooden box and mounted it on three skates. One skate was fastened on each side and the third in the center back to serve as the rudder. Then he had added a mast and sail. Everyone wanted to try skimming over the frozen river. Hans was busy all afternoon giving rides to his friends.

Many of the young men went home from that January afternoon on the river thinking, If Hans Schmidt can build an iceboat, why can't I? Within a few weeks there were more iceboats on the Hudson River.

Where and when did iceboats get their start? We will never know for sure. But it undoubtedly was in northern Europe, where winters were cold and boats were in common use. The people around the Baltic Sea, such as the Latvians and the Dutch, all had "sailing sleighs" at an early date. Often runners or skates were merely mounted under a sailboat for use in the winter. A Dutch painting made in 1768 shows a typical sailing boat with a crossplank running under the hull. A runner was attached to each end of the crossplank and a skate had been fastened to the bottom of the boat's regular rudder.

The Dutch settlers of New York State started making iceboats to sail on the frozen Hudson River in 1790. The sport gradually spread up and down the river. By the middle of the nineteenth century, it was very popular. Shortly after the close of the Civil War, the first ice yacht club was formed. By 1881 iceboating on the Hudson had taken on

142

an international flavor. At regattas held there, ice yachts from all over the world raced.

At this time the sport of iceboating was dominated by the wealthy. Rich owners built huge ice yachts that were handled and raced by professional crews. Extra crew members served as ballast and shifted their weight to control the iceboat when it rose on one runner. From the safety and comfort of their clubhouses the owners watched their ice yachts compete.

Typical of the ice yachts of this time was the *Icicle.* It was owned by Commodore John E. Roosevelt, uncle of Franklin D. The *Icicle* was 70 feet long and carried over 1,000 feet of canvas. Such yachts were the fastest vehicles of their day. The only things that could even approach them in speed were trains. The boats competed not only with each other but with trains. The tracks of the New York Central ran parallel with the Hudson River. The yachts raced the trains and usually beat them.

Iceboats can reach several times the speed of the wind if the pilot sails across the wind instead of allowing the boat to be pushed directly ahead of it. The *Scud* was clocked at 107 miles per hour in 1885. The *Clarel* was clocked at 140 miles per hour in 1907. It would be years before airplanes and automobiles equaled these speeds.

After 1900, the center of iceboat activity shifted to the rivers in New Jersey, and especially to the Midwest. There it flourished on the large inland lakes of Michigan, Minnesota, and Wisconsin.

The boats in use then were of the Hudson River type. They consisted of a single fore-and-aft spar—called the backbone. A wooden crosspiece, called the runner plank, was mounted across it. Runners were fastened to the ends of the runner plank. The steering blade, controlled by a tiller, was mounted under the stern end of the backbone. The mast with the sail was also mounted on the backbone.

ICEBOATING TODAY

About 1931, a new type of iceboat was developed in Milwaukee. This new design had the steering runner at the bow of the boat instead of the stern. The runner plank was moved to the rear. This new design was easier to handle and faster. It defeated all competitors. A smaller version of this design, known as a skeeter, was built. This boat soon became very popular. It was light, easy to transport, and capable of speeds of over 100 miles per hour. Today this is by far the most popular iceboat.

Iceboats and sailboats are handled in almost the same way. The principles are the same. Crew members lean their bodies going around turns to change the center of gravity and keep the boat from capsizing. The big difference between a sailboat and an iceboat, though, is the speed. For

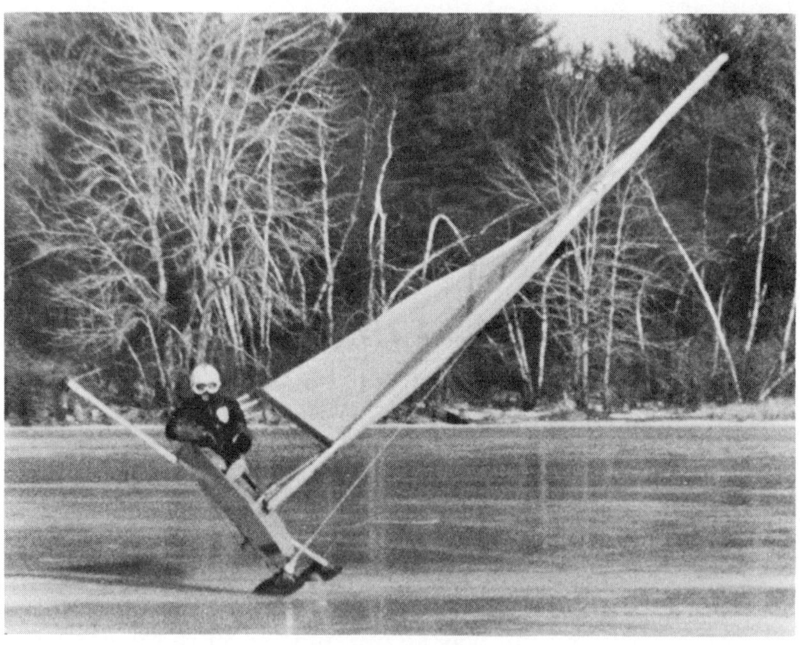

An iceboat "hiking"

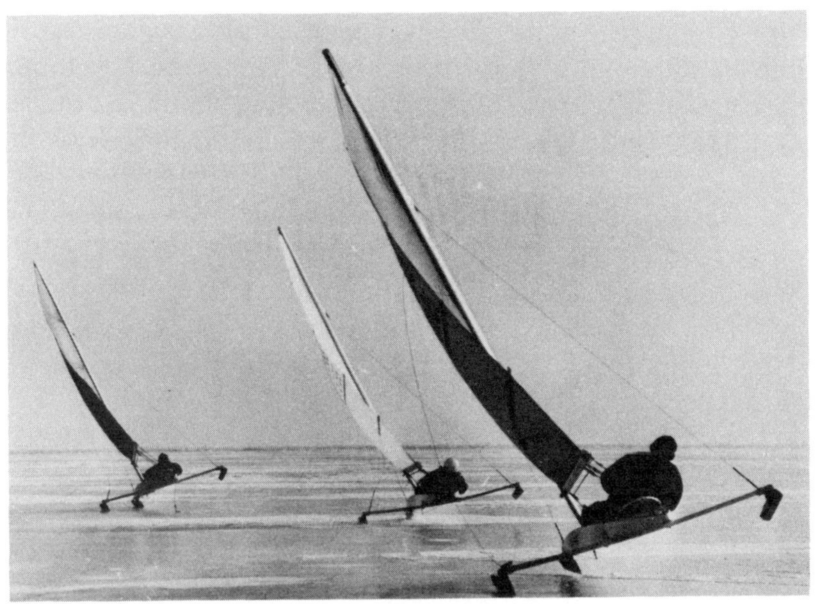

Iceboating should never be done alone

a beginner to jump into an iceboat and take off without any lessons is as dangerous as jumping into an airplane and taking off. A crash in an iceboat going 100 miles per hour can be as deadly as an airplane or automobile crash at that speed. Drivers are strapped in and wear crash helmets. But, other than that, they have no protection.

The most exciting part of iceboating is "hiking." This happens when the sail catches a sudden puff of wind. One runner rises off the ice. An expert pilot can glide along on one runner for about half a minute at fantastic speeds. But unless the pilot eases out on the sail and brings the runner down, there will soon be a high-speed crack-up.

There are, at present, no schools where you can learn to pilot an iceboat. (Iceboaters prefer the term "pilot" rather than "driver" or "skipper.") If you want to learn, go out where iceboats are sailing. Help the pilots and watch what they do. Offer to go along as ballast or crew while you learn

145

how to handle a boat. The beginner should spend at least one season doing this before he or she ventures out alone. The first trips on an iceboat of your own should be made in a light wind. It takes an expert to handle an iceboat in a brisk wind.

Iceboating, like scuba diving, should never be done alone. Out on the ice anything can happen. Always do your iceboating in a group, or with at least one other boat. Always remember that iceboats require a lot of open space. They cannot be operated safely around ice skaters and those engaged in other winter sports.

Many iceboats are homemade. Magazines sometimes publish plans for building an iceboat. One can usually be made for about $100. Kits to make one yourself can be purchased for about $500. If you are really interested in iceboating, you should write to an iceboating association near you. If you live where winters are cold, look in the yellow pages of the telephone directory for the name of one. The association will send you information about iceboating and tell you where supplies can be purchased.

12. SAND YACHTS

SAND CARS

Maurice of Nassau, the Prince of Orange, was giving a picnic. The courtiers clustered around the prince buzzed with excitement. Everyone hoped for an invitation. This would not be an ordinary picnic. The guests would travel in sand cars.

On a lovely morning in June 1600, forty courtiers, dressed in brilliant court finery, arrived by carriage at a beach on the North Sea. Servants loaded down with baskets of food and wine accompanied them. Other servants carried cushions for the guests to sit on. The courtiers murmured excitedly when they saw the sand cars lined up ready to take them on the jaunt.

The Netherland sand car had been invented a few years earlier by Simon Stevin, the Dutch mathematician. Sand cars were large, clumsy, creaking wagons on which square-rigged sails had been mounted. When the brisk winds from the North Sea blew from the right direction, the sand cars could roll along the beach at a speed of 25 miles per hour. This was by far the fastest speed of any vehicle at that time. Everyone was eager to enjoy this new thrill.

Twenty-six guests were seated in the largest sand car. The others rode in the smaller ones. Then they were off, rolling along the packed sand beside the North Sea. Sometimes they passed through the shallow water left by the retreating waves. The ladies screamed as the spray flew.

A secluded spot in the sand dunes was selected for lunch. Tablecloths were laid on the sand and cushions arranged around them. There the courtiers sipped wine and picked at fowl and fruit. The picnic was declared a huge success. Many of the guests predicted that horses would soon be obsolete. Everyone would depend on the wind for transportation.

But sand cars did not replace horses. In fact, there were not many places where there was enough space or wind to operate the bulky vehicles. Since the sails were fixed, the cars would only roll when the wind came from directly behind them. Carriages had to be sent out to pick up the courtiers on this picnic. The wind wasn't blowing from the right direction for them to return by sand car. But rolling over the sand was fun.

SAND YACHTS TODAY

Today land yachts—or sand yachts, as they are now called—are making a comeback. They are very similar to ice yachts and are sometimes referred to as rubber-tired iceboats. They do not offer much comfort. Sand yachts, like iceboats, have no springs. The movement of the springs would absorb too much of the wind power. Some sand yachts do have rudimentary brakes. One model has a hinged stick that can be dragged in the dirt to slow the car down. The sail on a land yacht is about the same as the one used on an iceboat. Both types are operated like a sailboat. Some land yachts have a steering wheel. Other lightweight models have a pedal that turns the front wheel. Most have three rubber-tired wheels, with sand tires being optional. On the beach these machines can attain twice the speed of the wind, or about 60 miles per hour.

A small sand yacht is not very expensive. Lightweight models, weighing about 70 pounds, sell for around $500. Builders of sand yachts have borrowed some of the concepts and materials used in hang gliders. Today the builders use aluminum tubing for the frame and dacron for the sail. The sand yachts can be disassembled or assembled in minutes, and folded up and carried on a car top.

The ideal place to enjoy a sand yacht is at the beach. But if there isn't a beach within a hundred miles of where you live, don't give up. Any smooth, open space will do. Bonneville Salt Flats is a favorite spot for wind racers. Hundreds of miles of smooth salt make it an ideal place for land yachts. At certain times of the year, when the salt flats are too windy for anyone else, land sailers take over. Shopping center parking lots are also good places for land yachts. Of course, you will have to schedule your trips for early in the morning or late at night.

There are clubs for land yacht enthusiasts all over the world. These hold races and rallies. Let's take a look at one of the most exciting sand yacht rallies ever held. In February 1967, the first Trans-Sahara Sand and Land Yacht Rally was held. This was the first mass crossing of the Sahara under sail. Twelve cars set out to travel seventeen hundred miles through Algeria and Mauritania. The trip took thirty-two days and only eight cars completed the trip. Sand, rocks, and the driving winds took a toll of cars and drivers. The drivers stopped counting flat tires after passing five hundred. Those who finished had rebuilt their land yachts several times. The route was chosen because the northeast wind blows twenty-six days of the month during the winter. With this wind behind them, the pilots were able to travel the seventeen hundred miles with no other power.

13. SAIL SKATING

OUTSKATING THE WOLVES

It was almost dark when Bernadette left the one-room schoolhouse on the edge of the deep woods. Evening came quickly in winter in the Province of Quebec. It would be dark by 4:30 P.M. Bernadette had stayed after school that day to clean the blackboards and erasers for Mademoiselle Du Fail. She had become so engrossed in her work that she had forgotten how quickly it got dark. Now the children she usually skated home with had all gone. The ten-year-old hurried down to an inlet of the frozen river and put on her ice skates. Then she hung her boots around her neck, picked up the lard pail, which served as her lunch bucket, and her kite-shaped sail. Quickly she was off down the inlet to the main body of the river.

Saint Anne River served as a highway for the French Canadians. In the summer they traveled its length in their bateaus, in the winter on skates and in sleds.

The farm where Bernadette's family lived was nearly five miles upriver from the schoolhouse, and her legs carried her to and from school. But Bernadette didn't feel that this was a hardship. Almost all the children traveled that far to school—some farther. It was easier to get to school in the winter. In the Province of Quebec, children learned to skate

150

almost as soon as they learned to walk. All skated to school in the winter. Most of them carried a sail to help them travel faster on the ice. Bernadette used an old sail that had once belonged to her brother, Jacques.

A full moon was rising as Bernadette set out for home. She made long sweeps with her old-fashioned skates. When she got out of this inlet, surrounded by trees, there should be enough breeze for her to use her sail.

When Bernadette got out to the main body of the river, she glanced back up the inlet. In the gathering dusk, she noticed a dark form slinking along near the trees. Idly she wondered what a dog was doing out there on the ice at that time of day. Bernadette adjusted her lunch pail and raised the sail between herself and the wind. A steady breeze was blowing up the river. It shouldn't take her long to get home.

Bernadette loved sail skating. The sensation of flying over the ice was exhilarating. In spite of the gathering darkness, Bernadette felt happy and only a little lonesome. Traveling at this speed, she had to watch the ice in front of her carefully. It was difficult to see the rough spots in this light. Bernadette began to sing "Alouette" at the top of her lungs as she flew over the ice. The song made her forget that it was almost dark, that she was alone and far from home.

Sch-r-r-r-r-u-u-u-n-n-n-c-c-c-h-h-h-h! Bang! Bernadette's lunch pail skooted across the ice with a big clatter. Her sail skated along in a different direction. Bernadette was down on her hands and knees. She hadn't seen that ridge of ice in the dim light and had plowed into it. She stood up slowly and, by the light of the rising moon, examined her knees. Her mother would be very cross with her. She had torn the knees out of another pair of stockings.

While Bernadette was gathering up her lunch box and the sail, she heard the first howl. *Oo-o-o-o-o-oh-h-h-w-w-w-w-w!* It came from over on her right. Bernadette glanced that way but saw nothing. Almost at once it was answered from down the river. *Oo-o-o-o-h-h-h-h-h-w-w-w-w-w-w!*

Bernadette looked back down the river. The moon made a dazzling white path on the frozen river. Several dark shapes were loping down this path toward her.

When Bernadette fell, she had been warm from her skating. Now she felt as if she had been dunked in the icy Saint Anne. Bernadette was a child of the north woods. She knew without a doubt that wolves were on her trail.

This was the middle of February. The winter had been long, cold, and cruel. All wildlife had suffered. The deer had all moved farther south, looking for food. Wolves had moved down from the north. At night Bernadette had seen them slinking around the farmhouse looking for a chicken or duck that had not been safely locked up for the night. No one at home went out after dark without a lantern.

Bernadette didn't hesitate. She knew she had only one chance. She got her sail in position and off she went again. Luckily the wind had picked up. Bernadette flew faster and faster. Desperately she peered in front of her, trying to avoid the rough places on the ice. She became conscious of a panting and clicking. She glanced back and to her left. There was a large gray wolf running all out, trying to catch up with her. But he was losing ground. She glanced to her right and saw another gray shape loping along. Bernadette was afraid to look back. She knew the rest of the pack was following her.

Bernadette knew the wolves couldn't catch up with her unless she fell. She was probably going 30 miles an hour. But what would happen when she got to the farm? It sat back on a knoll about two hundred feet from the river. She couldn't run fast enough on her skates and she wouldn't have time to put on her boots. If only she could get far enough ahead of the wolves so they couldn't catch up with her then.

Bernadette rounded the last bend a short way from her home. She took a quick look in back of her. About twelve wolves were stretched out behind her. The closest one was at least a hundred yards away—not far enough.

Two dark figures appeared on the ice in front of Bernadette. For a moment she couldn't take that in. Were the wolves in front of her too? Then she heard someone calling, "Bernadette! Bernadette!"

"Père! Père!" she called. "The wolves are after me."

One of the figures raised a rifle. The *crack!* echoed up and down the river. As if by magic, the wolves melted into the darkness. Bernadette's father and brother had been worried because she was so late getting home. They had come looking for her.

Could a little girl really sail skate faster than wolves could run? Well, people have been clocked at 50 to 55 miles per hour while sail skating. Wolves can't run that fast. There is an old Canadian legend that says a little girl did outskate the wolves one night on a frozen river.

SAIL SKATING LONG AGO

Sail skating, or skate sailing, probably appeared shortly after skates were first invented. When was that? A long time ago. Prehistoric bone skates have been found in Sweden that were made sometime between A.D. 800 and 1000. The first mention of ice skates in literature was in the reign of King Sigurd I, who died in A.D. 1130. At that time skates were made from the long bone of the foreleg of a reindeer. The bone was ground down until one edge was sharp. A couple of holes were bored through the bone so it could be tied onto the shoe. Later, skates were made of iron.

When all travel was by horse or on foot, it is not surprising that people eagerly seized upon any means of traveling faster. For a seafaring people, where great stretches of water were frozen in winter, it was quite logical to add a sail with skates. With a large sail, speeds of 30 to 40 miles per hour could be achieved, even on the primitive skates.

Sail skating undoubtedly originated in the Scandinavian countries and is one of the oldest sports. But its popularity has gone up and down. At times everyone was doing it, and at other times sail skating was forgotten. In the 1890s, members of a London skating club took up this sport and it became very fashionable in England. Early settlers brought the sport with them to Canada and the northern part of the United States. Around 1900, everyone was sail skating. It became common for children in the colder regions to sail skate to and from school.

HOW TO SAIL SKATE

Sail skating is one of the least expensive of all sports. All it takes is a sail and ice skates. For that reason it has always been popular with children. Almost anyone can fashion some sort of sail. The sail can be triangular, rectangular, or kite-shaped. The frame can be made out of bamboo or other lightweight wood. Muslin, hemmed on all sides, can be used for the sail, although balloon silk or dacron is better, because it is lightweight and stronger. The sail should be perfectly flat and the cloth stretched tightly. There is now a commercial sail on the market made with aluminum tubing.

One other thing is necessary before you take to the ice —warm, wind-resistant clothing. In sail skating, the wind does the work as it pushes you around. You are not very active, and the wind provides an additional chill factor. You will be warmer if you wear layers of clothing. Air is trapped between the layers to act as insulation. There is another advantage. When the sun comes out, you can remove a few layers. If you are planning on sail skating in a brisk wind, a crash helmet should be worn.

In sail skating, the sail is always held between you and the wind. A little knowledge of sailing is a big help. The sail

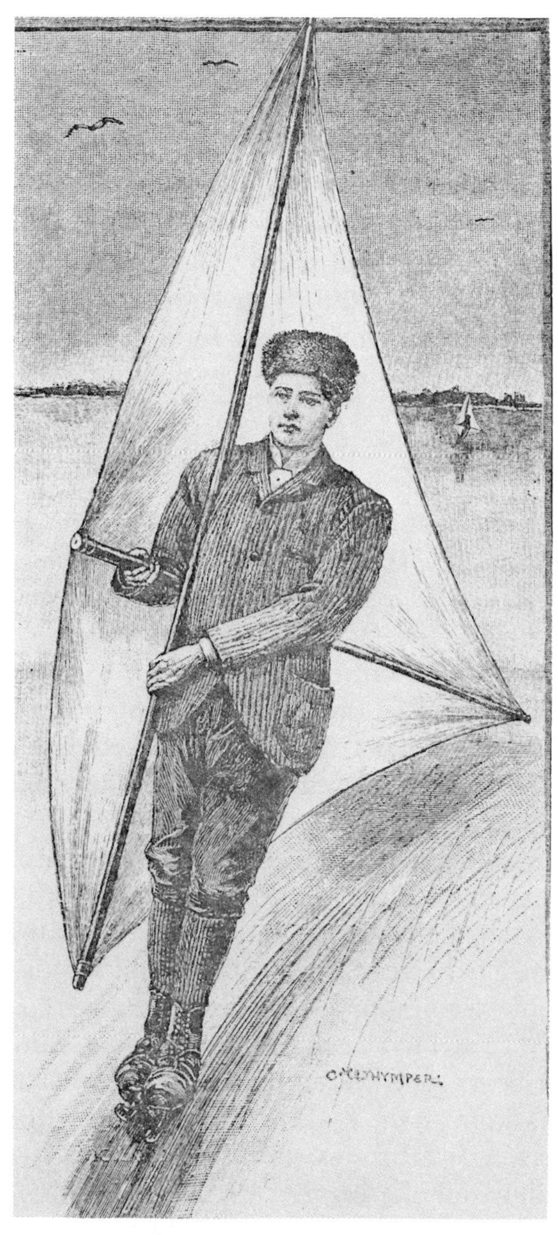

Sail skating about 1900

is used just as it is in a sailboat. When you want to turn or stop, the wind is spilled from the sail by raising it over your head. To "come about," or tack back against the wind, the sail is brought down on the other side of your body. Experiment a little and you will soon find out how the position of the sail affects the direction and speed at which you travel.

Most sail skaters find it isn't worthwhile to try to tack back against a stiff wind. You should always carry your boots hung around your neck. In sail skating, you never know when it will be easier to put on your boots, roll your sail, and walk back.

One of the big attractions of sail skating is that it is not necessary to be an expert skater to enjoy it. Only basic proficiency in skating is necessary. The sail gives stability and bears much of the skater's weight. Beginners should try sail skating first in a light breeze and with a small sail. The larger the sail, the faster the speed. It takes practice to master high-speed sail skating.

All sailers speak of the feeling of flying while sail skating. They don't feel as if their feet are touching the ice. This takes a little getting used to. But the experience is very exhilarating.

To be done safely, sail skating, like iceboating, requires a wide expanse of clear ice. Sail skaters don't have the control over their movements that ice skaters do. You should always be ready to drop the sail if it is taking you into trouble. Some sails have straps or cords to be used for fastening the sail to the skater. This is very dangerous. The sail can't be dropped in an emergency. Sail skating should always be done on the buddy system. Skate with at least one other person at all times.

Although sail skating has been in a decline for several years, it now seems to be making one of its periodic comebacks. Those who do hang gliding and sailsurfing in the summer have found they can use the wind for sail skating in the winter. You won't hear much about sail skating until

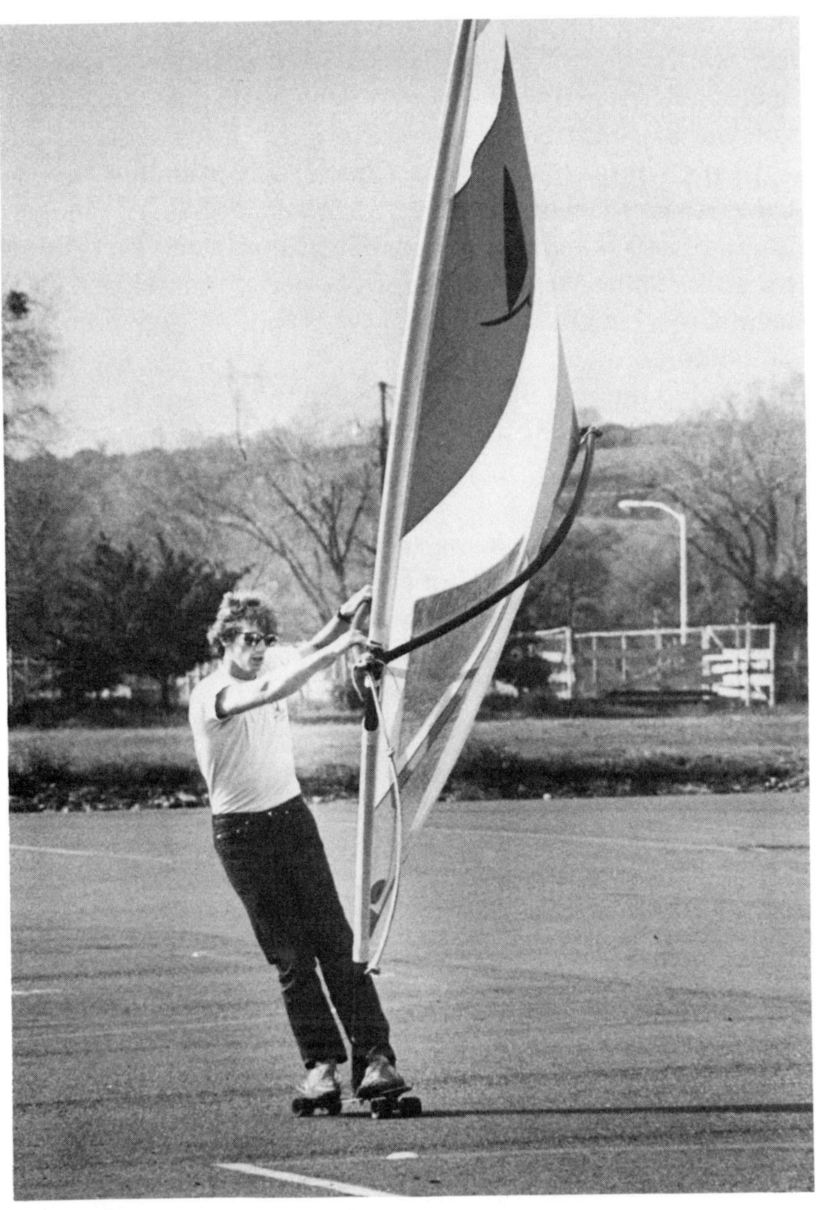

Sail skating on a skateboard

there is a big freeze. Then, where there is a large body of ice, someone will remember sail skating. A sail can be fashioned in a couple of hours or less. Then, add skates and you too can participate in an exciting winter sport.

In the winter of 1977, the Charles River at Boston was frozen from the dam to Harvard University. As if by magic, flocks of sail skaters appeared. They were using everything for sails. Some were made out of sheets and ski poles attached to a backpack frame. But everyone was out enjoying sail skating.

Would you, too, like to experience the sensation of flying without ever leaving the ice? If you would, the next time there is a cold snap in your neighborhood, remember sail skating.

Sail skating is also being tried on roller skates. Here the problem is finding a wide-open, smooth space. Parking lots or an abandoned airport runway or road are the only places that offer enough room for roller sail skating.

GLOSSARY

ACCURACY CONTEST   An event in which parachutists try to land on or near a target.

AERODYNAMICS   The science of the way air affects a body in motion.

AIRFOIL   Any surface, such as a wing, designed to aid in lifting.

ALTIMETER   An instrument to record altitude.

ANGLE OF ATTACK   The angle at which the leading edge of a moving airfoil meets the air.

ATTACHED TYPE OF PARACHUTE   A parachute fastened to the outside of the airplane or balloon.

BERNOULLI'S PRINCIPLE   The law stating that the pressure of a fluid or gas decreases when the speed of either one increases.

BIPLANE   An aircraft with two wings.

CATERPILLAR CLUB   A club whose members must have saved their own lives by jumping with a parachute.

CONTROL BAR   A bar on a hang glider used to control up and down movements.

DAGGERBOARD KEEL   A piece of wood that is dropped through a slot to provide more stability on a sailboard.

DRAG   The force that opposes the movement of a body through the air.

EJECTION SEAT   A seat that can be shot away from a disabled aircraft.

ELEVATOR   A hinged surface that controls the up and down movements of an aircraft.

FIXED WINGS   Wings that do not move.

FLAG FALL   A fall in hang gliding signaled by the flapping of the wing.

FLYING SPEED   The speed at which lift overcomes the force of gravity.

FREE FALL   A jump in which the jumper pulls the rip cord.

Free flight   Flight not held back by ropes or wires.
Gantry   A tower or framework.
Glider   A motorless heavier-than-air craft.
Glide ratio   The distance a craft travels forward for every foot it
   drops in still air.
Glider port   A landing field for gliders.
Hang glider   A glider in which the body of the pilot hangs down.
Heavier-than-air   Weighing more than air.
Hiking   In iceboating, sailing with only one runner on the ice.
Hydroplane   An airplane equipped with pontoons to enable it to
   land on water.
Internal-combustion engine   An engine in which fuel is burned
   inside the cylinders.
Jibbing   Sailing with the wind.
Keel boom   A post or rod down the center of a sail to provide
   stability.
Leading edge   The edge facing the direction of motion.
Lee wave   A rapidly flowing stream of air that blows over a moun-
   tain, hits the ground, and rebounds.
Lighter-than-air   Weighing less than air.
Manned flight   A flight carrying a person.
Motor-driven winch tow launcher   A device for launching a
   glider by towing it to the edge of a cliff.
Mountain wave   A rapidly flowing stream of air that blows over a
   mountain, hits the ground, and rebounds.
Parascending   Same as parasailing. Using a lifting parachute be-
   hind a speedboat.
Powered flight   A flight with an engine.
Prevailing wind   In a given area, the direction from which the
   wind usually blows.
Ridge lift   The lift provided when the prevailing wind hits a cliff or
   hill and is deflected upward.
Rigid-wing glider   A glider with stiff wings unable to bend.
Rip cord   A handle and cord used to open a parachute.
Rogallo wing   The cloth wing invented by Francis Rogallo now
   used on most hang gliders.
Rudder   Device used to control left and right movement of an air-
   craft or boat.
Sailplane   A light, streamlined glider.
Segmented wings   Wings divided into parts.
Shock-cord launcher   A device for launching a glider by snapping
   it off a cliff.

160

SHROUD LINES   The lines that run from the parachute canopy to the harness worn by the jumper.

SINKING SPEED   The distance a craft travels forward for every foot it sinks in still air.

SKY DIVING   A parachute jump with a long free fall.

SOAR   To fly by using an updraft of air.

SPOT-LANDING CONTEST   An event in which the jumpers try to land on or near a target.

STABLE POSITION   A position used by parachute jumpers—belly down, back arched, arms and legs extended—to keep from tumbling.

STAGE RACE   A race made in legs or steps.

STATIC LINE   A line attached to an aircraft that pulls the parachute from the bag and starts its deployment.

STRATOSPHERE   The region that extends from 11 to 30 miles above the earth.

STREAMLINING   Shaping a body to offer less resistance to air or water.

STYLE EVENTS   Jumps where turns and loops are performed during free fall.

TACKING   Sailing against the wind.

TETHERED   Fastened to the ground by ropes or cables.

THERMAL   A column of rising warm air.

TRIPLANE   An aircraft with three wings.

ULTRALIGHT   Very light glider equipped with an engine.

VARIOMETER   An instrument to measure whether an aircraft is rising or sinking.

WARPING   Twisting.

WIND METER   An instrument for measuring wind speed.

WIND TUNNEL   A pipe in which air is blown past a model to test aerodynamic design.

WISHBONE BOOM   An elongated, elliptical boom that goes around the sail on a sailboard.

BIBLIOGRAPHY

BOOKS

Bixby, William. *The Hang Gliding Book.* David McKay Co., 1978.

Canby, Courtlandt. *A History of Flight.* Hawthorn Books, 1963.

Crouch, Tom D. *A Dream of Wings.* W. W. Norton & Co., 1981.

Dwiggins, Don. *Bailout.* Crowell-Collier Press, 1969.

Emrich, Linn. *The Complete Book of Sky Sports.* Macmillan Co., 1970.

Flower, Raymond. *The History of Skiing and Other Winter Sports.* Methuen, 1977.

Flying Magazine, Editors of. *Sport Flying.* Charles Scribner's Sons, 1976.

Greenwood, James R. *The Parachute.* E. P. Dutton & Co., 1964.

———— *Parachuting for Sport.* Modern Aircraft Series. Sports Car Press, 1962.

Halacy, Dean. *Soaring.* J. B. Lippincott Co., 1972.

Harris, Sherwood. *The First to Fly.* Simon & Schuster, 1970.

Hart, Clive. *Kites.* Frederick A. Praeger, 1967.

Knight, Clayton. *The Story of Flight.* Grosset & Dunlap, 1954.

Liebers, Arthur. *A Complete Book of Winter Sports,* rev. ed. Coward, McCann & Geoghegan, 1971.

Lucas, John. *The Big Umbrella.* Drake Publishers, 1973.

Penzler, Otto. *Hang Gliding.* Troll Associates, 1976.

Peterson, Gunnar, and Edgren, Harry D. *The Book of Outdoor Winter Activities.* Association Press, 1962.

Radlauer, Ed. and Ruth S. *Racing on the Wind.* Franklin Watts, 1974.

Rice, Herman. *True Flight.* True Flight, 1972.

Richards, Norman. *The Complete Beginner's Guide to Soaring and Hang Gliding.* Doubleday & Co., 1976.

Sellick, Bud. *The Wild, Wonderful World of Parachutes and Parachuting.* Prentice-Hall, 1981.
Woodward, Richard, and Sheffield, Robert, eds. *The Ice Skating Book.* Universe Books, 1980.
Yolen, Jane. *World on a String.* World Publishing Co., 1968.

MAGAZINE AND NEWSPAPER ARTICLES; BULLETINS

Colligan, Douglas. "Hang Gliding." *Science Digest,* June 1976.
Dee Boucher, Gen. Jean. "Dry-land Fleet Sails the Sahara." *National Geographic,* Nov. 1967.
Hamilton, Mildred. "Hanging Out There." *San Francisco Examiner,* Nov. 20, 1977.
Hawkes, Russell. "Happy Birthday, Otto Lilienthal." *National Geographic,* Feb. 1972.
James, Stuart. "How to Ice Skate on a Sunfish." *Popular Mechanics,* Feb. 1979.
Kocivar, Ben. "Land-sailor You Can Car Top." *Popular Science,* Feb. 1979.
McKeown, Bill. "Hottest Thing Under Sail." *Popular Mechanics,* May 1981.
Newman, Bruce. "It's a Bird, It's a Plane." *Newsweek,* Mar. 23, 1981.
Record Searchlight, Aug. 8, 1981. "Wind's Up."
Soaring Society of America. *Soaring in America.* (No date.)
Sunset Magazine, Feb. 1971. "You Can Watch, Ride or Take Lessons."
Sunset Magazine, Aug. 1981. "Windsurfing."
U.S. Hang Gliding Association. Various bulletins.
Wahl, Paul. "A Whole New Breed of Hang Gliders." *Popular Science,* May 1974.
Woodings, Paul. "Go Fly a Big Kite." *Times/Outlook,* May 18, 1977.
Young, Gordon. "Sailors of the Sky." *National Geographic,* Jan. 1967.

INDEX

ABOUT THE AUTHOR

ANABEL DEAN, an elementary school teacher for more than twenty years, has written numerous science books for young people. She is a graduate of the State University of California at Arcata, California. The mother of three, she resides in Redding, California.